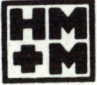

THE NURSE AND THE WELFARE STATE

SERIES EDITOR
June Clark BA MPhil SRN HVCert

In the same Series

Professional Responsibility in the Community Health Services
Health Education – Practical Teaching Techniques
Counselling and the Nurse – An Introduction
Hard-to-Help Families
Infant Feeding and Family Nutrition
Sociology for Community Nurses
Multiple Births

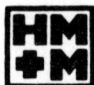

HM+M TOPICS IN COMMUNITY HEALTH

The Nurse
and the
Welfare State

Edited by

JEAN GAFFIN BSc(Econ) MSc
Organising Secretary, Child Accident Prevention
Committee, London; Formerly Senior Lecturer in
Social Policy, Department of Nursing and Community
Health, Polytechnic of the South Bank, London

Contributors

JUDITH ALLSOP CertEd BSc(Econ) MSc
JEAN GAFFIN BSc(Econ) MSc
LESLEY RIMMER CertEd BA MSc
KATE ROBINSON BA SRN HV

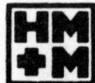

HM+M H M + M PUBLISHERS
Aylesbury · Buckinghamshire · England

First edition, published by
H M + M Publishers Ltd, Milton Road,
Aylesbury, Buckinghamshire, England

0 85602 089 3

Contributors

JUDITH ALLSOP CertEd BSc(Econ) MSc
Senior Lecturer in Social Policy
Department of Social Sciences
Polytechnic of the South Bank
London

JEAN GAFFIN BSc(Econ) MSc
Organising Secretary, Child Accident Prevention Committee
London; Formerly Senior Lecturer in Social Policy
Department of Nursing and Community Health
Polytechnic of the South Bank, London

LESLEY RIMMER CertEd BA MSc
Research Officer, Study Commission on the Family
London; formerly Senior Lecturer in Economics
Polytechnic of the South Bank, London

KATE ROBINSON BA SRN HV
Research Assistant, Department of Nursing
and Community Health Studies
Polytechnic of the South Bank
London

Typeset by Dolphin FotoType, Aylesbury, Buckinghamshire
Printed in Great Britain by A. Wheaton & Co. Ltd., Exeter

Contents

Preface   vi

Glossary of Abbreviations   viii

1 Social Policy: Who Decides?   1
Judith Allsop Jean Gaffin

2 What do we mean by the Welfare State?   20
Judith Allsop

3 Parties and Politics   33
Jean Gaffin

4 Paying for Services   46
Lesley Rimmer

5 Did Poverty Die when the Welfare State was Born?   61
Lesley Rimmer

6 The National Health Service   81
Judith Allsop

7 The Personal Social Services   116
Judith Allsop

8 Housing   136
Jean Gaffin

9 Nurses and the Welfare State   147
Kate Robinson

Recommended Further Reading   160

Useful Addresses   161

Index   163

Preface

This book is for all nurses. Why should nurses be interested in the welfare state? Firstly, as users of the social services: such use is obvious when a child goes to school or a grandmother draws her old age pension. Equally obvious is central and local government involvement in the provision of council housing, but less obvious is government aid to house buyers through tax relief on mortgages. Nurses are users of these services in just the same way as other citizens.

Secondly, as taxpayers and ratepayers. Decisions about whether one social service will grow whilst another shrinks; what is the right balance between unemployment benefit and the average wage; should the elderly be more generously treated ... these decisions affect our pocket, and we need to be aware of the way such decisions are made.

Thirdly, nurses work in one of Britain's largest industries, in terms of money spent and the number of people employed. To influence policies within the National Health Service, an understanding of the economic and political context of health care, and its relationship to other social service provision is essential. As nurses become increasingly aware of their ability to influence decisions about how health care is delivered, this kind of knowledge will be even more vital.

Lastly, but not least, nurses in hospital and in the community are consulted by patients about a wide range of problems. An understanding of the provisions which exist to help to meet some of these needs, and knowing what professional and what statutory and voluntary agencies might help, is an important part of the knowledge of a helping and caring profession. Nevertheless, this book discusses issues and principles rather than providing a comprehensive description of every service available: for this, readers are recommended to read the three books listed under Essential Reading on page 159 which describe health and social service provision in detail, including that provided by the voluntary sector, and are revised regularly.

JEAN GAFFIN

1981

Note The proportion of women admitted to medical schools is rising, and more men are being attracted into general nursing — but overall, most doctors are men and most nurses are women. If nurses are referred to as 'she' in this book it is not because we wish to perpetuate sex-role stereotyping but for the sake of simplicity and as a reflection of reality.

Acknowledgement

The heaviest cost when working married women take to writing books is borne by their families: less shared time, ever scrappier meals and a general increase of bad temper. Thank you!

JUDITH ALLSOP
JEAN GAFFIN
LESLEY RIMMER
KATE ROBINSON

GLOSSARY OF ABBREVIATIONS

ACAS	Advisory, Conciliation and Arbitration Service
AHA	Area Health Authority
ANO	Area Nursing Officer
CHC	Community Health Council
COHSE	Confederation of Health Service Employees
DHA	District Health Authority
DHSS	Department of Health and Social Security
DMT	District Management Team
DNO	District Nursing Officer
FPC	Family Practitioner Committee
GDP	Gross Domestic Product
GNP	Gross National Product
GP	General Practitioner
HAS	Health Advisory Service
NALGO	National Association of Local Government Officers
NHS	National Health Service
NUPE	National Union of Public Employees
PESC	Public Expenditure Survey Committee
RAWP	Resource Allocation Working Party
RCN	Royal College of Nursing
RHA	Regional Health Authority
RNO	Regional Nursing Officer
SB	Supplementary Benefit
SBC	Supplementary Benefit Commission
SSD	Social Services Department
TUC	Trades Union Congress

Chapter 1

Social Policy: Who Decides?

Judith Allsop   Jean Gaffin

Who makes policy in Britain? How is it made? Who decides how much money will be spent on health services? Or whether family planning services will be free of charge? Or whether services for the mentally handicapped should have higher priority than renal dialysis units? Or whether a particular hospital should close? Or whether health visitors should be 'attached' or geographically based?

What influences these decisions? How do policy makers decide between alternative strategies? And how can we – whether as individuals, or as voters, or as workers in the health and social services, or as members of organisations – ensure that such decisions are what we would wish?

To answer these questions we must understand something about political processes and in particular how these processes operate in Britain. There are many conflicting views – one reflection of this is the large number of books on the subject. In studying the institutions which make policy at both national and local level, however, there are two main approaches. The first is the formal approach which emphasises the constitutional framework of government, looking in particular at Parliament, the Cabinet and the role of the Prime Minister. The second approach lays greater emphasis on the reality of power as exercised 'behind the scenes', for example by pressure groups of various kinds. The role of the media is important also to this approach, especially as elections come to be fought from the television screens rather than by door-to-door canvassing.

The perspective taken in this book follows the second approach and is pluralist in emphasis; that is, it assumes that policy emerges as a result of conflicting pressures. Central government sets the scene, with financial constraints and policy objectives. Local authorities develop very different patterns and levels of service which reflect local political interests, local needs and local community pressures.

1

Social policy defined

In discussing the welfare state, the term social policy is often used. The term is usually taken to mean central government and local government activities concerned with providing *services* (ie. health, education, housing and social services), or *income* (ie. social security benefits) for its citizens. *Social* policy is closely linked with *economic* policy. Tackling rapid inflation and high unemployment involves economic policy, but trying to cope with the stress and hardship that follows is a task for the social services – so completing the circle.

Social policy is about how much welfare the state should provide, how it should be paid for, and who should get what – and how. Reaction to these questions depends on political views and attitudes, discussed in Chapters 2 and 3 of this book. We may argue about social provisions in this country but we recognise that social policy is about *benefits* in cash or kind. However, social policy is not always benevolent. Hitler's Germany had a social policy towards gipsies and the mentally handicapped that led to the mass murder of these groups (along with other groups, of which the largest, by far, was the Jews). The USSR often sees opposition to the State as 'mental illness', and uses its psychiatric hospitals to contain opponents of the regime. (Amnesty 1975).

Chapter 4 considers how we pay for social services. That chapter reminds us that WE pay: you and I. As a relatively low-paid profession, nurses are not big contributors in absolute terms, but if we consider the amount which is contributed to the state through general taxation (eg. income tax) and on purchases, as well as to the National Insurance Funds and to rates, the nurse may well feel that a disproportionate amount of her income is spent by other people on her behalf. It sometimes comes as a surprise, therefore, to realise that in international terms we are taxed more lightly than many other nations. For example, Britain comes 11th out of 18 in the world league of industrial countries in terms of the proportion of our national income which is collected in tax (Economic Trends 1979). But because Britain collects a larger amount through income tax, rather than through taxes on expenditure, the British taxpayer *feels* more highly taxed than others living in industrialised countries.

The social services

We might begin by reminding ourselves that compared with some other countries we are not particularly big spenders as far as social services are concerned. If we take expenditure on health services, for example, and look at how much other countries spend per head of population, we find that in 1974 Britain spent £88 per head, compared with £146 by France and £173 by Sweden (adapted from the Report of the Royal Commission on the NHS 1979).

The major social services provided by the welfare state are:

social security
health services
education services
housing services
personal social services.

These social services, provided by central and local government, are not the only way in which social needs are met. The informal network of support provided by family, friends, neighbours and colleagues is also important, helping *far more* people than the statutory services. There is a wide range of voluntary organisations, varying from the small self-help group (eg. of widows in one small town) to a large, national voluntary organisation such as Barnardo's, which provides a great deal of residential care and community help to children and families in need.

In addition, there is commercial and private provision of social services, such as the privately-run homes for the elderly or mentally handicapped, as well as the individual child minder. Private provision usually flourishes when statutory services are inadequate. The insufficiency of places at local authority day nurseries has led to the rapid growth of child minding. Rising hospital waiting lists are one factor in the increasing use of private medical insurance schemes. Long waiting lists for local authority homes for the elderly create the demand for privately-run homes.

How policy is made   In order to understand the social service provisions explained in detail later in the book, it is important to understand how central government and local government work, how decisions are made, and the influences which affect them.

Central government

After an election, the leader of the party which has obtained the most seats is invited by the Queen to form a government. He (or she) becomes Prime Minister and chooses a group of members of parliament from his own party to work closely with him: most of them will be in the House of Commons, but some may be in the House of Lords. On rare occasions (eg. in times of war, or when there is no clear majority), members of the government may be chosen from other parties as well, thus forming a coalition government. The government is composed of ministers and others given responsibility for particular areas of policy. These ministers and junior ministers are responsible for the work of government departments. At the Department of Health and Social Security (DHSS), junior ministers are responsible for the separate spheres of policy within the department: social security, health and social services. They are members of the government, along with the Secretary of State for Social Services who is politically responsible for all the activities of the DHSS – but only the Secretary of State is a member of the *Cabinet*. The Cabinet is the key decision-making body of the government: it is a committee of senior ministers, under the chairmanship of the Prime Minister, which formulates policy and makes the most important decisions, eg. about the legislation that will be brought before Parliament, the extent of public expenditure, and so on.

The Secretary of State for Social Services and his junior ministers are responsible for the decisions that are made *within* the DHSS, but other matters, especially when they relate to major changes of policy or where finance is involved, will be referred to the Cabinet for decision. In the Cabinet, the Secretary of State for Social Services has a dual role: he represents the interests of the DHSS but he is also a member of the Cabinet, playing a full part in the making of collective decisions about government policy. Richard Crossman, when Secretary of State for Social Services, faced this dilemma in January 1969: he had to spend much time fighting inside Cabinet for a pay recommendation for doctors which the Prices and Incomes Board opposed as they thought it to be inequitable and inflationary (Crossman 1977).

The Secretary of State for Social Services and his ministers are supported by a large staff of some 5,000 civil servants. Some of them are concerned with policy, and some with the levels of service and with questions of how services are best provided. The civil servants in the DHSS are drawn both from the professions (eg. nurses, doctors, pharmacists) and from the lay, career Civil Service. Professional staff include the Chief Medical Officer and the Chief Nursing Officer.

Civil servants will tend to stay with the DHSS for a number of years, although changing jobs within that Department, whereas ministers may change quite often – and not just because of elections, but also when governments are 'reshuffled' as, for example, following a resignation or a changing emphasis within the government.

Although policy decisions are formally made collectively by the Cabinet as a whole they are the product of both internal and external influences. The party in power in Parliament, the size of its majority, the views of the national party organisation, public opinion, the views and style of a particularly strong minister, the strength of the views of senior civil servants and, above all, the strength of the Prime Minister – all can affect policy decisions.

If the Cabinet is the central point of decision making, there may be small groupings of senior ministers from the Cabinet who are influential, as shown in the recent diaries of former cabinet ministers (Crossman 1977; Castle 1980).

Ministers bring to the Cabinet proposals for discussion which may, if accepted, become government policy, but may, of course, be rejected! Proposals may come from the party's election manifesto, or be suggested by civil servants. Governments have considerable power in deciding how existing policies are modified and implemented: this may not require *new* legislation, as most existing legislation contains scope for change and modification. The amount of money devoted to the National Health Service can be changed without prior reference to Parliament, although Parliament will be told later about the changes. The Cabinet plans the programme of legislation for the parliamentary year and determines the order in which such legislation will be taken, but the views of the party, junior ministers and backbench members of parliament will be taken into account. A new government usually begins its legislative programme by trying to implement some of the ideas contained in its election manifesto (eg. the Housing Act 1980, discussed in Chapter 8).

The Prime Minister is the formal head of government and is usually seen as the most powerful member of the Cabinet. It is likely that the priorities and interests of particular prime ministers will affect particular areas of policy (eg. Edward Heath was strongly in favour of Britain joining the Common Market, James Callaghan initiated the Great Debate on Education, and Mrs Margaret Thatcher's views on monetarist economic policies have dominated policy making in her government). The fact that the Prime Minister appoints *and* dismisses the members of the ministerial team inevitably affects the balance of a government. The Prime Minister must make sure, however, that the Cabinet represents the various shades of opinion to be found within the political party concerned.

Health and social services are rarely of great philosophical concern to the Cabinet, but the DHSS is one of the highest-spending departments and this is where its importance lies when policy is being considered. This is one reason for the inclusion of the Secretary of State for Social Services in the Cabinet, which began when Richard Crossman was given that post in 1968.

Cabinets make the final decisions but the ground is prepared for Cabinet discussion by Cabinet Committees, which are also important. Cabinet committees and ministers are in turn supported and briefed by senior civil servants. It is frequently argued that the higher levels of the civil service, particularly in the Treasury, have considerable power and influence over policy making in Cabinet and it is perhaps for this reason that ministers have begun recently to appoint political assistants to keep them in touch with attitudes within their own party, and so balance the civil service view.

In the creation of policy, the Treasury has a special role: to evaluate policy proposals in terms of cost-effectiveness and in terms of the implications for future spending. More recently, the Treasury has been most concerned with restraining public expenditure. The Treasury's attitude towards policy is influential at every level of policy making: *within* departments, and in Cabinet discussions. Indeed, in Cabinet the Chancellor of the Exchequer, who is the political head of the Treasury, is one of the most influential of ministers.

A crucial factor in the power of government within the House of Commons is the size of its majority. A rebellion by backbench MPs over a certain issue (eg. the revolt in 1980 over payment for school transport) is more important when the government has a *small* majority. The Labour government maintained a majority in the House of Commons from 1977–1979 only because it was supported by the votes of Liberal MPs, which forced the Labour government to modify some of its policies (eg. the 1978 budget). Social policies are decided by government and Cabinet, but they are frequently based on ideas generated from outside, for example, by pressure groups; these ideas are discussed and evaluated within government departments before they reach the Cabinet.

A further and crucial general influence on policy making is the concern shown by all governments, starting in the 1960's, but continuing through the 1970's and into the 1980's, about the lack of growth in the economy, the high rate of inflation and growing unemployment. Governments since the war, as we will see in later chapters, see economic management as one of their most important functions. Control of public expenditure is part of this task. Strategies have varied but this does not alter the fact that central control of public expenditure now plays a large part in economic policy and so has come to dominate social policy.

Nurses will be aware how difficult it is for radical changes to take place within the NHS. The management structure is cumbersome, public expectations are high, and the service is the centre of much pressure-group activity. These issues will be discussed in further detail in Chapter 6, but these constraints are important to the discussions throughout the book – above all in a period when public expenditure on the NHS is being relatively reduced.

Pressure groups and policy making

Parliament, and particularly the House of Commons, can be seen as a forum in which much, if not all, pressure-group activity takes place. Pressure groups, or interest groups, are groups of people who have a strong common interest which they wish to promote. They try to influence government policies but (unlike a political party) are not interested in taking power themselves.

There are two major kinds of pressure group. Firstly, there are the *protective groups*: their purpose is to defend the interests of their members. Examples of this kind of group include the Automobile Association which seeks to defend the motorist, and the trade union which seeks to protect its membership in the same way as the employers' federation protects its members. Examples of protective interest groups in the health field include the Confederation of Health Service Employees, the Royal College of Nursing and the British Medical Association.

The other main type of pressure group is *promotional*: seeking to promote a cause through a wide appeal to the general public to back up its pressure on Parliament. The Child Poverty Action Group promotes the cause of the poor, as the Royal Society for the Protection of Animals promotes the cause of animals. In the health field, the Patients' Association seeks to promote the cause of the patient, and the Disablement Income Group that of the physically handicapped.

The ease with which members of pressure groups can get their case heard by civil servants or MPs differs. The fact that those who speak for industry tend to have easier access is important. For example, the strength of the tobacco interest or the alcohol industry is greater than that of, say, the anti-smoking lobby, or of doctors running clinics for alcoholics, *despite* the costs to the NHS of the continuing level of tobacco and alcohol consumption.

Party activists and constituency lobbies as well as pressure groups use MPs to promote their interests. MPs, in turn, have a number of ways of influencing the government. They can apply pressure on Ministers, promote debates in Parliament and initiate Private Member's Bills (eg. the Chronically Sick and Disabled Act 1970 started life as a Private Member's Bill initiated by Alfred Morris). Parliament is certainly taken seriously by ministers and their departments.

In addition, there are Parliamentary Select Committees where small groups of MPs from all parties investigate and review particular aspects of policy. The two major long-standing select committees are the Public Expenditure and the Public Accounts Committees. Since November 1979 there have been 14 additional select committees of MPs relating to 14 different government activities, one of which considers the work of the Department of Health and Social Security. These committees have power to question the Secretary of State and junior ministers, as well as civil servants from the Department, on a wide range of matters. Pressure groups, especially those with factual information to offer, may also be asked to give evidence to these Select Committees.

Pressure groups in the health and social services

Groups representing medical interests are perhaps the most influential in the health and personal social services. The Royal Colleges, the British Medical Association and the General Medical Council provide membership for departmental committees, advisory bodies and committees of enquiry. MacKenzie (1979) refers to this group of 60–80 doctors as a 'political class'. As well as providing membership for this kind of committee, such organisations are also active in *promoting* the interests of their members within the DHSS and in Parliament. There are also a number of more vocal but less influential organisations, such as the Junior Hospital Doctors Association, who may take the centre of the stage on certain issues such as pay and conditions of service. Organisations such as the Royal College of Nursing play the same role on behalf of nursing, but although nurses are a more important group numerically, their organisational strength does not yet match that of the medical profession. However, when legislation was finally introduced in Parliament in 1979 (following the Briggs Report of 1972), the original proposals were substantially amended following pressure-group activities by midwives and health visitors.

It is often through Parliamentary pressure that Committees of Inquiry are set up. Such Committees investigate particular incidents (eg. the death of Maria Colwell), or particular issues (eg. family violence). There is often general agreement that a problem exists but lack of agreement about how to resolve it. In these circumstances, a Royal Commission or a departmental or inter-departmental Committee of Inquiry may be a useful way of dealing with a wide range of problems. Interest groups, although giving evidence to the Committee or the Commission, may participate and influence decisions and recommendations.

The extent to which action follows the Reports of such Committees varies. Sometimes a report leads to rapid implementation of a recommendation, or to legislation (eg. the Seebohm Committee Report 1968 led to the Social Services Act 1970). Other reports, despite presenting a fascinating and detailed picture of a problem, achieve very little in terms of concrete proposals. An example of a particularly interesting and thorough Committee Report which was followed by relatively little action was *Fit for the Future* (Court

Report 1976), which examined in detail needs and provisions in the child health services. For nurses the most important recent report was that of Briggs (1972), entitled *Report of the Committee on Nursing* (Chairman: Asa Briggs), which made detailed proposals for the education of nurses and a number of other recommendations about the future of nursing.

The professional organisations which represent nurses in government circles include the Royal College of Nursing (RCN), the Health Visitors Association and the Royal College of Midwives, which are the old-established professional associations and negotiating bodies. Most of the professional associations are now also certified trade unions, but nursing membership of all trade unions has been growing rapidly during the last few years. The Confederation of Health Service Employees (COHSE), started as the union for nurses working in mental hospitals, but now represents a wide range of hospital workers, as well as an increasing number of general nurses. The National Union of Public Employees (NUPE) recruits a wide range of ancillary hospital workers and some nurses. The growth of trade unions within the NHS, and growing nurse membership, is an important aspect of the changing NHS, the changing influences on it, and the changing atmosphere in which the nurse works. The role of these organisations is discussed in more detail in Chapter 9.

The main professional organisation for social workers is the British Association of Social Workers, which recently set up a separate trade union, the British Union of Social Workers. As most social workers are employed by local authorities, the National Association of Local Government Officers (NALGO) remains the most important trade union for social workers. Other local authority staff employed in social service work may belong to NUPE, and the Residential Care Association is also relevant. Pressure groups representing professional and occupational workers are but one kind of group attempting to influence government policy, as has already been shown.

Many pressure groups, are concerned to promote particular kinds of policy or simply to improve existing services for particular groups of people, and so span both health and social service department provisions. For example, MIND (National Association for Mental Health) and the Disability Alliance are nationally-based organisations which comment and put forward views on policies affecting the client groups (the mentally ill and the physically handicapped) whose interests they promote. In addition, MIND has local Associations for Mental Health under its wing which keep an eye on local needs and provisions and may sometimes be involved directly in providing some facilities for the mentally ill.

Pressure groups, including the professional ones, use the media to give publicity to their views (specialist journals as well as the national press, radio and television). Government departments regularly circulate cuttings files to their staff. How effective any pressure group is depends on a wide variety of factors, not least the links which the leadership have with top-level civil servants and senior politicians. The work of Eckstein (1960) and Willcocks (1967) shows the influence of different groups of doctors on policy changes within the health service.

Until recently there was little evidence that a 'public opinion' existed in relation to health service policy in general. As the public expenditure cuts introduced by the Labour Government in the late 1970's and by the Conservative government in the early 1980's took effect, local campaigns against bed and hospital closures won widespread local support. One possible explanation for the initial general indifference towards national health policy could have been the belief that the major issue of health service provision was resolved in 1948 with the introduction of a health service free at the point of consumption.

Local government

The ability of central government to see that its policies are carried out by local authorities is an important aspect of explaining the pattern of provision of social services, especially if we seek to explain why services vary so widely from one local government area to another. The structure and functions of local government need to be understood, and a brief description follows. It is hoped that readers will want to find out more about their own local area and its policies, in which case their town hall will be a useful source of information.

Local government is responsible for about one quarter of all public spending, hence its importance in economic as well as in political terms. In the 1970's, about 60% of local government expenditure was met by central government through the Rate Support Grant. The remaining expenditure is financed mainly from rates, with small amounts collected in charges. In the eighties, the proportion of local finance coming from central government is decreasing, leaving local authorities with *stricter controls* over the total amount they spend but *fewer controls* over the way they spend the money they have allocated to them by central government.

Policy decisions within local government are made by groups of elected Councillors, and in deciding policy they must be aware of the costs that will fall directly on the ratepayers. As the ratepayers are the very people that have voted these councillors into office, there is often tension between the desire to provide a better service and the fear that the costs of that service (ie. increased rates) will make the councillors unpopular with the electorate. This contrasts with the situation within the NHS, where those who make the policy decisions are generally appointed by the Secretary of State for Social Services, and most of the cost of the NHS is met from general taxation. When making decisions that increase costs, the NHS managers are therefore divorced from the kinds of financial and electorial pressures which may influence local councillors. However, they must work within the cost limits set by the DHSS.

Central government controls the amount which local authorities can borrow for capital projects and this is nearly as important as its control of the size of its financial grant. Local government can act only when central government passes legislation that enables it to do so. Some Acts are *mandatory*, ie. they tell local authorites that they MUST do something (eg. provide education for all children between the ages of 5 and 16). Other legislation is *permissive*, ie. local authorities MAY do something if they choose to do it (eg. they may provide as extensive a library service as they like). In addition to legislation, government Circulars (formal letters sent to all relevant local authorities), although lacking the sanctions that legislation entails, usually do lead to local government compliance, as will be discussed in Chapter 3.

Less attention has been given here to the effects of pressure groups at local level than at central government level. Interest groups and promotional groups do also exist at the local level. Some of the pressure can be negative (eg. a pressure group of residents who are anxious to prevent the siting in the area of a hostel for men discharged from prison). There is also positive pressure (eg. from parents of mentally-handicapped children for improved facilities). National pressure groups often have local branches, eg. Age Concern and the Child Poverty Action Group. Other local groups are concerned with environmental issues rather than social problems. It is important to note that clients of the Social Services Department, as the most vulnerable members of the local community, are less likely to form pressure groups than, say, those organising to prevent new housing in their area or protesting against a new road scheme.

Summary of the responsibilities of the principal councils. (From the Local Government Handbook, *published by the Labour Party and reproduced here with its kind permission.)*

RESPONSIBILITIES OF PRINCIPAL COUNCILS

There has been a tendency since the second world war for local government to lose some of its responsibilities to governmental or ad hoc agencies. This tendency has been reinforced recently by the setting up of separate health and water authorities which came into operation at the same time as the new local government structure. On the other hand, local authorities have, since the war, also acquired new or expanded responsibilities in many fields, including the personal social services, planning, transportation, and the operation of the Community Land Act.

The present allocation of functions outside London is:

ENGLAND
County Councils (outside Metropolitan areas) and
Metropolitan District Councils

Education
Youth employment
Personal social services
Libraries

All County Councils

Museums and art galleries*
Housing
  Certain reserve powers

All District Councils

Museums and art galleries*
Housing
  Provision
  Management
  Slum clearance
  House and area improvement

Town development*
Planning
Structure plans
Development plan schemes
Development control in
certain areas
Derelict land*
National parks
Country parks*
Conservation areas*
Building preservation notices*
Tree preservation*
Acquisition and disposal of land
for planning purposes, de-
velopment and redevelopment*
Footpaths and bridleways
Surveys
Creation, diversion and ex-
tinguishment orders*
Maintenance
Protection*
Signposting
Transportation
Transport planning and co-
ordination

Town Development*
Planning
Local plans

Development control generally

Derelict land*

Country   parks*
Conservation areas*
Building preservation notices*
Tree preservation*
Acquisition and disposal of land
for planning purposes, develop-
ment and redevelopment*
Footpaths and bridleways

Creation, diversion and ex-
tinguishment orders*

Protection*

Transportation

All County Councils

Highways
Traffic
All parking

Public transport (as PTA in
metropolitan counties)

Road safety
Footway lighting*
Environmental health
Animal diseases

Refuse disposal
Consumer protection

All District Councils

Off-street parking (subject to
county council consent)
Public   transportation under-
takings   (non-metropolitan
districts with Local Act powers
only)

Footway lighting*
Environmental health
Food safety and hygiene
Communicable disease
Slaughterhouses
Offices,   shops   and   railway
premises
Factories
Home safety
Refuse collection
Clean air
Building regulations
Coast protection
Cemeteries and crematoria
Markets and fairs

Police
Fire (including fire precautions under Offices, Shops and Railway Premises Act 1962)

Leisure services	**Leisure services**
Swimming baths*	Swimming baths*
Physical training and recreation*	Physical training and recreation*
Parks and open spaces*	Parks and open spaces*
Smallholdings	Allotments
	Local licensing
Airports*	**Airports***

* *Concurrent powers*

WALES

The distribution of functions is the same as for the non-metropolitan areas of England with the following exceptions:

(i)   Welsh district councils are responsible for both the collection and disposal of refuse.

(ii)   Welsh district councils may provide both off-street and on-street parking facilities with county council consent.

(iii) Welsh district councils may, by order, be designated the food and drugs authority and the weights and measures authority or the public library authority (in practice four district councils have been designated as library authorities).

GLC	**London Boroughs**
Town and country planning — overall planning	Education (except in the Inner London boroughs)
Roads — metropolitan roads	Housing
Fire services	Roads (but not Metropolitan roads)
	Planning — development control and local plans
	Social services
	Public health
Shops Acts	Consumer protection
Smallholdings	
Management of the stocks of houses owned by the former LCC, the London authority for new and expanded towns	
Art galleries, museums and entertainment	Libraries, art galleries, museums and entertainment
Parks, playgrounds and open spaces — power shared with the London boroughs	Parks, playgrounds and open spaces
Licensing	
Bye-laws	

N B Education in Greater London

The London Borough Councils outside the former LCC area, which is known as 'Inner London', are education authorities. In Inner London a special committee of the GLC, known as the Inner London Education Authority (ILEA) administers the service. ILEA may require the GLC to raise such funds (from rating authorities in the Inner Area) as it may determine. This is the ILEA precept.

The ILEA consists of the GLC councillors elected for Inner London constituencies together with one member of each Inner London Borough Council and one member of the Common Council of the City.

Social policy and the welfare state

More than half the population of Britain – all those under the age of forty – have no direct experience of life without the welfare state. Among the older generation, early experience may colour attitudes to the present system. In both groups, attitudes to the welfare state vary. On the one hand are those who would have us believe that public money is being squandered on those unwilling to work, that doctors are besieged by hypochondriacs and that the schools are turning out illiterates. On the other hand the welfare state also has its defenders. They remind us that poverty and social deprivation exist in Britain even in the 1980's. They would of course agree that life is better, for even the very poorest, than it was in the 1930's. The degrading poverty of the mass unemployed of the 1930's has disappeared. Working-class women no longer fear illness or even motherhood, as they did before the introduction of the National Health Service. The opportunities for working-class children to reach university and polytechnic and receive a degree-level education have grown, albeit slowly, since the last war. But many defenders of the welfare state would go on to argue that it is still not enough. We should be working towards a more equal and more just society, they would argue, using the contributions of those who can afford to pay them to improve the quality of life for the old, the sick, the disabled, the unemployed and the low-paid. In fact, both the 1979 and 1980 budgets which reduced public expenditure are likely to have had the opposite effect!

Supporters of the welfare state point not only to the differences between the richest and the poorest. They point also to the differences between the living standards of the average family and those of the poorer sections of the community. Freezers, cars, holidays, telephones and new clothes are a normal aspect of life for many families today. They are *not* the normal way of life for the growing proportion of the population who are low-paid, unemployed, disabled and old.

Later chapters in this book look in detail at such questions as what is the welfare state and what is poverty, as well as describing the structure and function of the health, social service, social security and housing provisions. This chapter is concerned merely to explain how the welfare state works – and that means how it works for all of us, whether defenders or attackers – with the hope that those on both sides of this debate will gain a clearer and more objective view of its operation.

Professionals, politics and social policy

There is a feeling among some professional groups, and particularly among nurses, that politics and caring for people just don't mix. This view is often expressed as a plea to 'take the health service out of politics'. The fact is, however, as the Royal Commission on the National Health Service (1979) has pointed out, that no service which takes such a large part of public resources can be 'taken out of politics' however it is financed or administered. Moreover, the Royal Commission went further: 'We do not believe that this is in any wider sense desirable. Obviously there are aspects of the nation's health which would be better left out of *party* politics, but we believe it is both inevitable and right that the affairs of the NHS should be kept firmly at the centre of the public debate' (para 19:10). Exactly the same could be said of the other social services which are discussed in this book.

Those, such as nurses, who work within the health and social services have a special interest in the way in which social policy operates in their services. We hope that the chapters on the NHS and Social Services Department will demonstrate this. The standards of provision, the morale of those working in the service, the availability of necessary equipment, the employment of sufficient ancillary staff, the satisfaction of client or patient – these factors must surely affect the way the nurse views social policies. Whether the nurse regards herself as an attacker, a defender or a neutral onlooker, the debates now raging on public expenditure and the welfare state are about the work-load and the working conditions of all those who are employed in the NHS and all those who use its services.

The political and social environment in which nurses (and other NHS personnel) work is different from that of social workers because of the different distribution of responsibilities between central and local government. Social workers are in many ways closer to decision making. They will know who is Director of Social Services and which councillors are members of the Social Service Committee of their local council. They may well participate in local political activity, pressure-group activity or in a ratepayers group. Nurses can make their voice heard through professional groups and trade-union activities at both national and local levels – and at the work-place. Some of these channels of influence are discussed in the final chapter of this book. But NHS policy-makers are not elected and so cannot be lobbied as directly as local councillors, and if lobbied may be less responsive than councillors whose position depends on the electorate rather than on a non-democratic system of appointment. From time to time the argument for a locally-elected health service is heard. It would make the NHS more democratic but the medical profession is totally opposed to the proposal and there is very little public pressure for this change. The effectiveness of all those working in the health and social services who seek change depends on their own awareness of where and how decisions are made – and their willingness to use that knowledge.

In the next chapter we look at definitions of the welfare state and what various writers on social policy believe the state should do for the welfare of its citizens.

References

Amnesty (1975) *Prisoners of Conscience in the USSR: Their Treatment and Conditions.* London: Amnesty International

Castle B. (1980) *The Castle Diaries 1974–76.* London: Weidenfeld & Nicholson

Crossman R. (1977) *Diaries of a Cabinet Minister, Vol. III.* London: Hamish Hamilton & Cape

DHSS (1976) *Fit for the Future. Report of the Committee on Child*

Health Services (Chairman: Professor D. Court) Cmnd 6684. London: HMSO

DHSS (1972) *Report of the Committee on Nursing* (Chairman: Professor A. Briggs) Cmnd 5115. London: HMSO

Eckstein H. (1960) *Pressure Group Politics*. London: Allen & Unwin

Labour Party (1979) *Local Government Handbook: England and Wales*. London: Labour Party

MacKenzie W. J. M. (1977) *Power and Responsibility in Health Care: the NHS as a Political Institution*. Oxford University Press

Royal Commission on the National Health Service (Chairman: Sir Alec Merrison) (1979) *Report*. Cmnd 7615 London: HMSO

Report of the Committee on Local Authority and Allied Personal Social Services (1968) (Seebohm Report) Cmnd 3703 London: HMSO

Willcocks A. J. (1967) *The Creation of the NHS*. London: Routledge & Kegan Paul

Chapter 2

What do we mean by the Welfare State?

Judith Allsop

Since the nineteenth century, governments in all industrial societies – Japan, the United States of America, Communist Bloc countries, Western European democracies – have been increasingly involved in providing social services for their citizens. There has been much argument about how much or how little governments *should* do in relation to welfare, and about how much they *can* do to meet particular needs or offset disadvantages. This chapter examines different ways of describing and analysing the concept of the welfare state. Ideas differ about the proper role of governments in providing welfare. These different ideas are explained in the first part of the chapter; in the second part, the general social changes which have led to the increase in social provision are discussed.

Definitions of the welfare state

Let us begin with Briggs' (1977) definition of the welfare state as '. . . a state in which organised power is deliberately used (through politics and administration) in an effort to modify the play of market forces in at least three directions'. These directions are '. . . the provision of a minimum income for all, the provision of income for specific "social contingencies" like sickness or old age, the provision of a certain range of social services'.

The definition perhaps needs one qualification. Part of the activity of modern welfare states has also been the attempt to modify *indirectly* the play of market forces through, for example, government management of the economy in the prevention of unemployment and attempts to create employment by various means, as well as through maintaining income and providing services.

The range of social services which is provided in most advanced countries includes social security, health, education, housing and personal social services. In addition to these major services, there is a range of services in the area of leisure and recreation which could also be called 'social services'. The boundary between what is and is not a social service is vague.

The welfare state's provision of income and services may not always come directly through central or local government agencies. Titmuss (1963) has made the important distinction between social services which are provided by the state and benefits which are received through employers or the tax system. Benefits provided by employers in addition to wages (such as pension schemes, help with school fees, or subscriptions to private medical care schemes) are described by Titmuss as *the occupational welfare system*. He also argued that the taxation system redistributes income from those without to those with children. Benefits that come from the tax system are known as *fiscal welfare* (eg. tax relief on mortgage interest or on private pension schemes), and are equally part of the welfare state. The interaction between these three types of welfare, ie. social welfare, occupational welfare and fiscal welfare, is highly complex but all three affect *who* benefits from welfare and *in what way*.

There are three major points of view on the role of welfare in society. One assumes that there are two 'natural' channels through which an individual's social welfare needs should be met: the family and the market economy. Families, for example, should look after their elderly relatives and young children. Wages should be earned by jobs found in the market. If the market and the family do not function adequately, the State may then act to provide a minimum degree of support. This idea of, or attitude towards, the welfare state has been given a number of labels, eg. a residual model of welfare, or the laissez-faire approach to welfare. The implication is that there are only minimum rights to welfare, of subsistence level; the obligations of the State and government are limited, and should be used only in the last resort. These ideas are generally associated with the political right wing.

The second major approach takes the view that industrialisation has brought profound changes which are beyond the ability of the individual to cope with or control. Therefore the State MUST take responsibility for certain aspects of economic management (eg. control unemployment) and social provision (eg. provide health care) but in a way which will enable individuals to help themselves. Further examples of this would be the provision of old age pensions or sickness pay through social insurance schemes which involve contributions from State, employee and employer. The State might also be involved in providing services such as certain education or health services where the wider needs of society justify collective provision: but for only as long as these did not interefere with individual liberties. This approach to the welfare state has been called the liberal or 'reluctant collectivist' view, and is associated generally with an approach to politics which is neither particularly right-wing nor particularly left-wing.

The third set of ideas is the collectivist approach, which is associated with left-wing politics and puts forward the view that in a complex modern society the individual cannot provide fully for himself and family, and the provision of a range of social services is 'normal'. In this case the State's role is two-fold: it is the agency through which a system of legal social rights to services is guaranteed, and it becomes the agency through which incomes, goods and services are transferred so that greater social equality is achieved. Titmuss's concept of the division of welfare, which takes into account occupational and fiscal welfare as well as the traditional social service provision, becomes essential to this definition of the welfare state, because it incorporates the *total* distributional effects of all systems of welfare.

These different views of the welfare state sum up particular clusters of opinion about the proper role of welfare. Any actual welfare state is likely to contain services, institutions and policies which approximate to all three of these views and there is often a middle ground between them. Nevertheless, they represent identifiable viewpoints in contemporary debates about the social services, and for this reason they are discussed in relation to the views of the two major political parties in Chapter 3.

A number of writers have argued that a welfare state is impossible without a welfare society, and that it is more important to focus on society than the state. It could be argued that it is the family, the work group, the social group which determines the individual's social position, life-style and quality of life to a greater extent than the distribution of income and the provision of services by any government. If there are great differences between the rich and poor of a society (ie. if the social structure is highly stratified), the extent to which a welfare state can compensate for disability, deprivation or inequality is strictly limited. It demands a more radical redistribution of wealth than social policy yet involves. The other important quality of social groups is the extent to which these are caring networks. If these do not exist it is then exceedingly difficult for the state to create them.

These difficulties tend to be stressed by those who take a critical and perhaps pessimistic view of the extent to which a welfare state can redistribute income and services. There are others such as Titmuss (1963) who have argued that the welfare state itself could create a welfare society. Titmuss believed that the provision of social services would help to draw together different groups in society. State services such as the NHS, by being available to all, help to integrate minority groups, and by providing the same treatment prevent the development of second-class services for second-class citizens. Other aspects of the NHS, such as the Blood Donor Service, provide an opportunity for an altruistic voluntary gift through which the individual expresses his involvement in, and commitment to, the community, thus strengthening the cultural bonds of the nation. These views represent an idealistic account of the possibilities of the welfare state (Titmuss 1970).

There is another sense in which the welfare state could be seen as a welfare society, and this is in the large numbers of people and organisations involved in providing welfare. The welfare state functions by means of a great number of specialised activities. Some of these are carried out by professional groups such as doctors, nurses and social workers, and others by government agencies employing administrative staff, as in social security offices. The welfare state in action takes the shape of an extremely extensive and complex set of special bodies. In addition, there are voluntary organisations which, even if partly maintained by public funds, have considerable control over the way they interpret problems and in the execution of policy. They occupy a middle ground as providers of services between the government (or controllers of resources) and those people in receipt of social services. The large number of people employed as providers form an important and growing group. Their relative job security and good working conditions contrast with the lives of many of those whom they are employed to help.

The views on welfare discussed so far in this chapter have, in general, stressed the benefits of the welfare state. Some radical critics of the welfare state reject this: Gough (1979) argues that welfare has developed as a means of maintaining the advanced capitalist state, and that capitalism needs to produce labour (through health and education systems) and needs to maintain consumer spending (through a limited amount of redistribution) so that the goods which the market produces are sold. Gough goes on to suggest that the present economic crisis in many western industrial societies reveals the inherent contradictions in their welfare states. Increasing levels of public expenditure are proving to be necessary to satisfy the needs and demands of the working class. There is corresponding unwillingness among higher income groups to pay for services in an economy which has ceased to produce high growth-rates. The result is a crisis in capitalism, centred on the welfare system.

Radical critics of the welfare state also emphasise the control aspects of welfare. The growth of professional welfare bureaucracies is seen as a growth in the numbers of people who can tell others what to do; for example, whether a person can or cannot have a council house, or can send his child to the school of his choice. These criticisms of the welfare state contain some truth. Welfare can bestow benefits *and* imply control. Sufficiently democratic institutions are needed to counteract these controlling tendencies (eg. the Community Health Councils discussed in Chapter 6.)

It is very easy to point to inadequacies in the welfare state. In many areas, as described in Chapter 3, the welfare state has failed to alleviate poverty or distress, and so achieve greater social justice. There are conflicts of interest about who gets what and who pays for what – which may affect powerful interest groups in painful ways. What is certain is that arguments about social policy reflect the tensions which these changes create. We now turn to the changes brought about by industrialisation, the development of the welfare state in Britain, and explanations for its growth.

The development of the welfare state

'Technological changes of industrialism lead to changes in the structure of society, these societal changes produce or intensify concern about certain social problems, which creates demand for welfare services'. This is how Wilensky & Lebeaux (1965) explain the origins and growth of state provision of welfare. Not all writers on the development of the welfare state would agree with Wilensky & Lebeaux's explanation of events, nor would they accept the smooth transition between them which suggests a rational and inevitable chain of events. But before looking at different views of the development of services, let us examine some of the changes which did occur in 19th-century Britain. Certainly, the form of social life in the family and factory, city and suburb changed as a result of industrialisation.

During the late 18th century large-scale production in agriculture (through the enclosure movement) and industry (through the factory system) began to increase. Neither of these modes of production was new, but it was their intensification and extent which brought change. By the mid-19th century Britain was the workshop of the world as the growing concentration of the work-force in mining, factory production and shipbuilding led to a relative decline in the number of those employed in agriculture. The expansion of communications and transport, together with the growth of industry and trade and the long period of foreign wars, encouraged the movement of the increasing population to urban and industrial areas. Cities and towns, with their suburbs, grew. The total population of Great Britain increased from 10 million in 1801 to 23 million in 1861 and to 37 million in 1901. In 1801, 49% of the population lived in urban industrial areas; by 1861 this had increased to 60% and by 1901 it was about 70% (Mencher 1968).

The major consequence of these changes, for the majority of individuals, families and their dependants, was a new dependence on wage labour as a source of economic security and a breaking of traditional forms of social and economic life such as the family group, the craft, the guild, and the parish. These networks of relationship were often broken by the move to towns where the reliance on a wage became, for most, the only form of subsistence. Many factors could interrupt the payment of wages: ill health, disability, old age, lack of (or irregular) employment, or the death of the wage earner. The level of wages might also be inadequate to meet a family's needs. In the early part of the century the vulnerability of the growing working population was increased by the lack of organisation and power in the labour movement. The insanitary conditions of towns and poorly-built homes contributed to this social distress.

It was not surprising that by the turn of the 19th century there was considerable intellectual and political debate about the relief of poverty and the role of government in alleviating distress. The Elizabethan Poor Law had placed responsibility for the poor, both the able-bodied and those unable to work, on the parish, and this system was placed under severe strain, particularly in certain areas, by the greater volume of poverty brought about by industrialisation.

The response of the first Parliament which followed the passing of the Reform Act 1832, which gave the vote for the first time to property owners, was the Poor Law Amendment Act of 1834. This Act is an important milestone in the history of social policy in Britain because it remained on the Statute Book until 1948 and because it so clearly represents the laissez-faire view of the State and the relief of poverty.

The new Poor Law in effect forced the relief of poverty back onto the traditional sources of support, such as they were, limiting the role of the State to the relief of paupers in the Workhouse. Jeremy Bentham argued that all government was a great evil, and was justified only when it increased social and economic individualism or on utilitarian grounds, ie. on the grounds of the greatest good for the greatest number. And if government acted to mediate in social relationships, then government must be efficient, so paradoxically the first central government institution for regulating welfare (The Board of Poor Law Guardians), was influenced by the spirit of laissez-faire.

The 1834 Poor Law established workhouses in which the conditions were to be worse than those of the living conditions of the lowest-paid labourer. Those who entered the workhouse lost certain rights and privileges; for example, the family unit was broken up, they became 'less eligible', they became, in effect, paupers, a particular class in society. The Poor Law was rarely operated with full rigour. Firstly, Bentham's notion of centralised efficiency was in many ways unworkable; for example, wages varied throughout the country so it was difficult to establish in practice the level at which to operate the workhouse test. Secondly, it proved difficult to treat paupers as one category. Medical Officers were increasingly appointed to care for the sick poor in separate wings of the workhouse or, in some places, separate buildings. Out-door relief was often given to groups such as the elderly or disabled as opposed to the able-bodied.

Laissez-faire ideas about poverty and the role of the state dominated 19th century attitudes in government and charity circles. By the 1890's notions of the social causation of poverty began to gain ground: it was not *always* the individual pauper's own fault! Charity in fact was seen by certain sections of the middle classes as the great regenerator of morality in the fight against poverty. As Octavia Hill put it to the Royal Commission on the Housing of the Working Classes, 'I am concerned with improving tenants, rather than improving houses' (Frazer 1973). Charles Lock of the Charity Organisation Society, an agency concerned with channelling help to the respectable poor, commented with a curious contemporary ring that there was a danger of the State 'becoming caterers-in-chief' for its citizens (Frazer 1973). Charity in the 19th century was seen as a more legitimate channel of assistance than the government. It was designed to encourage self-help, despite increasing unemployment and a falling standard of living for the working classes, created by market forces beyond the control of the individual to influence.

A number of factors encouraged a more general acceptance of the idea of the social causation of poverty at the turn of the century. The existence of social distress began to be more forcibly presented as the power of the labour movement increased through the organisation of trade unions and increased parliamentary representation. The thorough and convincing survey work of Booth and Rowntree, in East London and in York, underlined the social situation of those in poverty. The poor were the elderly, the unemployed, the sick, and those with large families or low wages (ironically it is these very groups that are most at risk of poverty in the 1980's). They were not necessarily feckless, as had previously been imagined, but they were *shown* to be the victims of circumstances beyond their control.

Economic theories were also changing, and there was greater recognition of the relationship between levels of employment and the fluctuations of the trade cycle. Added to changing perceptions was concern by the governing classes about Britain's hitherto internationally-dominant economic and political position, because terms of trade were turning against her as other countries became in-dustrialised. Recruitment for the Boer War revealed a low level of physical health in the general population. Behind all this lay a genuine and persistent fear among the middle classes of social revolution, and a knowledge that the Poor Law was failing to contain destitution; increasing numbers of people were on Poor Relief, and of these an increasing proportion were on outdoor relief.

The Public Health Acts of 1840 and 1875 and Forster's Education Act of 1870 were early examples of state intervention to promote what could broadly be called greater national efficiency. The sanitary movement was concerned with the prevention of ill health and the spread of disease through improvements in the sanitary conditions of towns. The authorities which were set up to provide clean water supplies, sewage, and refuse disposal systems were the precursors of local authorities as we know them.

The provision of a minimum level of education for the population was also seen to be necessary for a manufacturing country – other countries in Europe had led, Britain followed. Fears for national efficiency and competitiveness were stirred by the Boer War, which helped to make possible the extension of state education in the early 20th century, together with the establishment of the school health service and meals for school children – all areas in which parents had traditionally had sole responsibility.

The Fabians, the emerging Labour Party and later the Liberal Party put their weight behind increased state intervention through the provision of labour exchanges, minimal old age pensions and finally the National Insurance Act 1911 which established a basic insurance system for many manual workers for periods of unemployment and sickness.

These are the kinds of development on which the reluctant collectivist model of welfare is based. They represent state intervention as a means of offsetting some of the effects of the market economy, on a self-help principle. Large-scale unemployment and the depression of the 1930's created further economic and political pressure towards economic management and state services to provide minimum standards of living.

Contemporary thinking on poverty and the role of the State in welfare provision is discussed in later chapters. It remains now to return to the general explanations on why state intervention in welfare occurred in the way that it did during the 19th century and early part of the 20th century.

Consensus and conflict views of social change

We have already looked at the quotation from Wilensky & Lebeaux whose view was that welfare was an inevitable and necessary response to industrialisation. Much writing on social policy is in this vein. This type of explanation of social change falls into the category which sociologists call structural-functionalist theories. To illustrate – these theories explain the growth of public health institutions through the need of the state and of employers to prevent the spread of disease and so maintain a healthy workforce. Or in terms of family support, the argument might develop in the following way: modern industrial society requires a high degree of personal mobility for which the small nuclear family is best suited, but in the course of change new social problems are generated, eg. the elderly are left isolated, strains are imposed on young people, working married women experience conflict between their two roles. This in turn generates a variety of social services to deal with these very problems: old age pensions, welfare services, probation services, and so on. Society in effect is seen as an entity which responds to perceived needs.

Many of these theories also assume a *consensus* view of society: the notion that at a very general level societies have shared values and agree about the rules for resolving differences politically. Much of the language of social policy textbooks and government reports and documents is the language of consensus, and these works represent a search for answers to what are presented as commonly-perceived problems. For example, the Royal Commission on the NHS (1979) says 'we consider it legitimate and positively desirable to devote public resources to the maintenance and promotion of personal as well as public health, not only by the constraints of law, but also by offering exhortation, education and incentives'.

On the other hand there are those writers who stress the interests which are involved in promoting particular policies, or definitions of problems. Society is seen not as a system of consensus (where values are shared) but as a continually contested political struggle between groups with opposing goals and ideas about the world. George & Wilding (1976) put it in this way: '. . . the values of dominant social groups have been a major influence in social policy. What we loosely and uncritically call social values are, in fact, upper and middle class values legitimated by the institutional order and internalised by the whole population'. A number of consequences for interpreting the development of the welfare state follows from this view. Firstly, the amount of actual conflict in relation to particular policies tends to be understated. This comment was made at the Liberal Industrial Enquiry in 1928: '. . . there has hardly been one of the items of state action proved by experience to have been beneficient which was not hotly opposed at its inception as an unwarrantable invasion of individual liberty'.

Secondly, the role of vested interests in promoting particular types of solutions to problems is understated. To take examples from the development of medical care, professional groups in the 19th century began to establish control of the practice of particular areas of knowledge, not only in medicine and the law, but in architecture, nursing and the professional administration of the Civil Service. These groups had interests in supporting or more often in *preventing* certain kinds of development. There was increased demand in the first half of the 19th century for doctors with qualifications in general medicine, surgery and obstetrics, but the Royal College of Physicians and the Royal College of Surgeons fought all attempts to establish a general qualification in medicine (Varlaam 1979). It was not until the 1950's that a College (now the Royal College) of General Practitioners was established.

Similarly, there was considerable opposition from medical men to the development of nursing as a profession. Brian Abel Smith's fascinating account of the *History of the Nursing Professions* (1960) is couched in the terminology of the battleground as various interests vie for supremacy. Equally interesting is Jean Donnison's account of the growth of midwifery as a profession, *Midwifery and Medical Men* (1978), and Monica Baly's *Nursing and Social Change* (1973) also looks at this issue. New technologies were not readily introduced. There was often a great time-lag between discovery and general adoption. Lister's germ theory and ideas on aseptic surgery were first published in 1867 yet aseptic surgery was not in general use until the early 20th century.

The power of vested interests is developed a stage further by some writers who argue that the notion of class conflict is crucial in explaining whether or not social legislation is enacted, or is an influence upon the final form of legislation (Wedderburn 1965). However, many improvements in welfare legislation did follow, historically, the widening of the franchise to include larger numbers of the population.

The major aim of this chapter has been to indicate that accounts of welfare do differ, and that these accounts are often based on value judgements about man in society and the proper role of the state. This theme is developed in the following chapter, which examines different responses to changes in social structure, particularly demographic changes and changes in the structure of the family, which have influenced the growth of welfare provisions in the 20th century.

References

Abel-Smith B. (1960) *A History of the Nursing Profession.* London: Heinemann

Baly M. (1973) *Nursing and Social Change.* London: Heinemann

Briggs A. (1977) The welfare state in historical perspective. In Shottland C. (ed) *The Welfare State.* New York: Harper and Row

Donnison J. (1977) *Midwives and Medical Men.* London: Heinemann

Frazer D. (1973) *The Evolution of the Welfare State.* London: Macmillan

George V. & Wilding P. (1976) *Ideology and Social Welfare.* London: Routledge & Kegan Paul

Gough I. (1979) *The Political Economy of the Welfare State.* London: Macmillan

Mencher S. (1968) *Poor Law to Poverty Programme: Economic Security Policy in Britain and the US.* University of Pittsburgh Press

Royal Commission on the National Health Service (Chairman: Sir Alec Merrison) (1979) *Report.* Cmnd 7615. London: HMSO

Titmuss R. (1963) The social division of welfare. In *Essays on the Welfare State.* London: Allen & Unwin

Titmuss R. (1970) *The Gift Relationship.* London: Allen & Unwin

Varlaam C. (1979) *A Socio-legal Study of the General Medical Council.* Unpublished PhD Thesis. University of London (Bedford College)

Wilensky H. L. & Lebeaux C. N. (1965) *Industrial Society and Social Welfare*. New York: Glencoe Free Press
Wedderburn D. (1965) Facts and theories of the welfare state. In Milliband R. & Saville J. (eds) *The Socialist Register 1965*. London: Merlin Press

Chapter 3

Parties and Politics

Jean Gaffin

In the last chapter we looked at some of the ideas relevant to the development of the welfare state: in this chapter I should like to consider how these ideas are still important to the understanding of our own attitudes to various aspects of social service provision, and our interpretation of current social policies. These ideas lie behind the social policies proposed – and sometimes implemented – by the three major political parties which represent the mainstream of political thought in this country.

The 'reluctant collectivist' view discussed in the last chapter is closest to the policies of the Liberal Party. The laissez-faire approach dominates the policies of the Conservative Party, and the 'collectivist' view remains the dominant approach of the Labour Party. Despite these differences between the parties – and we shall look at some examples later in the chapter – Wilensky (1975) sees these ideological differences as of *political* rather than *practical* significance. He studied the public expenditure pattern of seven communist and seven capitalist countries, and found little difference in their expenditure on health and welfare services. He argues that left-wing governments often fail to *increase* social expenditure as much as they would like, and right-wing governments may not *reduce* it as much as they would like!

Wilensky explains this paradox by the changing demographic structure of all the countries studied: above all, by the increase in the numbers of the elderly, who are major users of the social security and health services, within the population of each country. He also suggests that the very provision of social services leads to greater demands and expectations from the general population.

Demographic change

Demography is the academic discipline concerned with population structure, which means the size of the total population, as well as factors such as the age structure, birth rate, marriage and divorce rate, sex ratio and so on. In this book we need only to consider the major demographic changes which are relevant to the health and social services.

The population of Great Britain has risen from 37 million in 1901 to 55·8 million in 1979. This continuous rise came to a halt in 1974, and 1979 showed the first population increase since then – due mainly to an increase in the rate of child-bearing. Within that population there is now a slight excess of men over women, the 'shortage' of women making it likely that there will be fewer unmarried women than ever before. It was women who, before the Second World War and just after it, formed the majority of nursing and social care staff.

The rising number of births each year and improved life expectancy has led to a significant increase in the number of elderly people: from 2·4 million in 1901 to 9·1 million in 1971 and to 9·6 million in 1977. This means that of every 100 people 14 will be elderly (ie. over 65), and produces a demand for social services that no government or political party can ignore, and has implications for family structure. In terms of the demand for welfare provision, it is estimated that over half the mentally disordered and the physically disabled people are elderly, and within these total numbers the very elderly, usually defined as those over 75 years of age, is the most rapidly growing group.

Two other demographic points need to be made; firstly, because divorce is now easier and cheaper one third of marriages involve remarriage for one or both partners; secondly, one family in ten has only one parent. Both factors have implications for the capacity of the family to look after its own dependants. Moreover, families are now smaller; in the 1870's two married women in three had five or more children – by 1925 the number of children was down to two.

The changing family

The links between the demographic structure and changes in the family are particularly clear if we look at the fact that the majority of elderly people now live alone. More married women, and more married working women, means fewer single women willing to care for their elderly relatives (Moroney 1976). Longer life-expectancy means that many of these 'younger' women are in fact elderly themselves. Moreover, a third of those over 75 years of age are childless, with a consequent reduction in the social contact and help available.

We have already noted that more women now marry: in 1931 26% of women would have been married by the age of 24 years, and by 1971 the proportion had become 60%. We have also noted that family size has fallen − in addition, married women begin their families at a younger age, and have their children in a shorter period than in earlier decades. The population is more mobile, relatives tend to live further away than at the turn of the century, and the family is more isolated than it was.

Young & Wilmott (1973) have an interesting approach to changes within the family: they trace the development of the family, starting from pre-industrial Britain where father, mother and children worked together in a simple, subsistence economic unit. They look next at the effects of the Industrial Revolution, where the husband is caught-up in the wage-earning economy, and finish with what they call the symmetrical family − this is seen as a home-centred nuclear family, where there is less segregation of roles and more equality, with both partners working inside and outside the home.

Women today are relatively free from the burdens of child-rearing, housework and financial dependency − thanks to contraception, labour-saving domestic equipment and to the increased importance of (and opportunities for) women at work. Yet the State finds it hard to move away from the view that a woman's place is at home, unless women are *needed*.

During the Second World War women were needed for the war effort. Day nurseries were therefore opened, but the number of day-nursery places declined after the war despite the growing importance of women to the economy. Yet it is important to remember that the number of families with incomes below the poverty line would *triple* if married women stopped working and that public expenditure cuts which reduce the working opportunities for women, (as do cuts such as those in the school meals service), will have implications for other parts of welfare provision. One could also argue that the State has still not come to terms with the need of the working mother to have her children cared for after school hours and during school holidays. Women, therefore, often work when their husbands are at home (eg. evenings and weekends), and these difficulties of child care may deter the single parent from working at all.

Demographic changes and changes in family structure (particularly in the role of women) are an important part of the background to the rapid development of social services during and after the Second World War.

The Beveridge Report

The Second World War involved practically the whole community. Never before had such a large proportion of the population been involved in the war effort nor suffered from its direct and long-term effects. Evacuation uprooted normal family life and disclosed the conditions in which the disadvantaged sections of the population lived. The war produced social unity, a feeling of national purpose and solidarity in the face of the enemy. The joint involvement of citizen and soldier in the war effort led to the idea that society after the war should be better for all, irrespective of class, creed or military status: as the whole resources of the nation were being employed during the war various social measures were taken which made it easier for the post war legislation. The 'equality of sacrifice' characteristic of the war effort was to be reflected in the 'equality of provision' which was MEANT to follow the post-war social legislation.

The hopes for post-war improvements came from the publication in 1943 of the Beveridge Report, the report of an interdepartmental committee set up by the then Coalition Government to consider the needs of post-war Britain. The Report looked at the range of social provision available and found it inadequate. The Report argued that there were five giants to be overcome on the road to reconstruction: Ignorance, Disease, Squalor, Idleness and Want. There were queues at the doors of His Majesty's Stationery Office when the Report was published.

The war had led to a demand for skilled workers of all kinds and had revealed gaps in the educational system, especially in technical education. The giant Ignorance was tackled in the Education Act 1944, designed to correct the deficiencies of the educational system, and to offer 'equality of opportunity' to all British children, with compulsory education from the ages of 5 to 15.

The giant Disease was tackled in the National Health Services Act 1946, which established a comprehensive health service for all, virtually free at the point of consumption and paid for mainly out of general taxation. The NHS is discussed fully in Chapters 6 and 9.

Squalor was, and is, a more difficult giant to deal with, especially as during 1939–45 there was no new building but only extensive bombing. But the war has a profound effect on post-war housing programmes, with a rapid development of council house building and emergency housing programmes, although demand grew much more rapidly than supply.

The giant Idleness was tackled in a White Paper on Employment Policy, published by the Coalition Government in 1944, in which the Government stated that they accepted as one of their primary aims and responsibilities the maintenance of a high and stable level of employment after the war. This was a major departure, but crucial, as unemployment had played the major part in causing poverty before the war and did so again in 1980.

But most important of all were the proposals for the giant Want. The Beveridge Report contained detailed proposals for a scheme of social insurance so that provision would be made to provide against interruption and loss of earning power, with incomes adjusted to family needs (ie. a system of Family Allowances was introduced). These and other parts of the legislation against Want are discussed fully in Chapter 5.

The National Assistance Act 1948, which was one of a number of measures against Want, also, in its Part III, abolished the Poor Law and introduced residential and community provision for the elderly, the disabled and the homeless. These provisions are discussed in Chapter 7, as are the services for children which were developed following the Children's Act 1948.

Published whilst the Coalition government was in power, the major legislation was passed in the life of the 1945–51 Labour Government. The early enthusiasm which followed the publication and partial implementation of Beveridge's proposals has declined. Some aspects of the welfare state are savagely attacked by the political right, yet the Labour government of 1974–1979 failed miserably to protect it from public expenditure cuts.

Let us now turn from the demographic and family context and the welfare state as it emerged after the Second World War to the rather different world of the 1980's.

British political parties

The nature of the British voting system encourages large parties. The Labour and Conservative parties in Britain contain a much wider spread of views and attitudes than you would find, for example, in much of western Europe, where parties are smaller, covering a narrower range of views, but then coming together into coalitions when a government is about to be formed. Our coalitions (apart from war-time) are found *within* our two major parties. The 'left' of the Conservative Party is sympathetic to improving social services. Similarly, the 'middle' and 'right' of the Labour party are convinced that a mixed economy is crucial as a safeguard for the individual liberty which has been eroded in such totally collectivised countries as the USSR. The 'right' of the Conservative Party is totally committed to a minimum of government interference; the Labour 'left' with the minimising of the role of capitalist enterprises.

The policies put to the electorate by the major parties, and often translated into action by the majority party that forms a government, reflect the major strands in British political thinking outlined in Chapter 1. But they are also the product of debate within each party.

The organising and financing of the political parties in Britain reflect their ideology and their supporters. Most of the finance for the Conservative Party comes, directly or indirectly, from large commercial enterprises. Most of the finance for the Labour Party comes from the Trade Union movement. Very few companies and no trade unions support the Liberal Party, and most of its funds come from the fund-raising efforts of its members. Members of the Labour and Conservative Parties also continually find themselves involved in fund-raising activities, but the money so raised provides a small proportion of the total finances of their parties (compared to the role such funds play in financing the Liberal Party).

When formulating policies, the two major parties are aware of the views of their major financial backers, as well as the social class and interests of the voters they are hoping to attract. Although health and social services are not as central to the concern of either the Trade Union movement or the business world as economic policy, the proportion of the country's wealth that is spent on such social services is a central and crucial part of economic policy, as is made clear in Chapter 4. One problem is that some of the profits from which large companies make their donations to the Conservative Party may be made by 'contributing' to ill health (eg. tobacco firms, companies selling alcohol).

Peter Calvocoressi (1978) suggests that social policy helps to keep the Labour Party *together* in spite of divisions about timing and pace, whereas the same social issues *divide* the Conservative Party, who are united on issues such as economic and industrial policy (on which Labour politicians tend to disagree).

The State, as shown in Chapter 1, has moved from doing as little as possible for those in need, to providing a basic minimum of services for the poor, the sick, the aged, the disabled and the young. Few Conservative voters would argue for dismantling the welfare provisions which we now have, but they are much more worried about the financial 'burden' of the care provided than the Labour voter is. As Calvocoressi argues, it is impossible to develop a welfare state without class conflict unless the national cake is growing bigger all the time. In a low-growth economy, the welfare state of a scope and quality that British people have come to expect conflicts with the fact that when the State meets the needs of those it decides to help, it intervenes to collect taxes from us all to pay for those services. To the political right, this suggests interference with personal freedom: to others, the scale and extent of poverty is a bigger problem than the obligation to pay taxes.

The modern political debate

The differences between the parties can be examined by considering the policies put forward in the 1979 election campaign. The central issue of that campaign was how to manage the economy, and so ensure economic growth and a slower rate of inflation. To the Labour Party economic planning was essential. To the Conservatives, reducing taxation in the hope of increasing investment was crucial. The 'lost' taxation was to be found by cutting public expenditure, with more emphasis on the market solution to social problems. Both parties made clear their commitment to reduce inflation, a problem easier to solve within the covers of an election manifesto than in the real world. What did they propose?

The Conservatives argued for strict control of the money supply, reductions in government borrowing and public expenditure, and measures to reduce direct taxation, and increased taxing of expenditure instead. In fact, one of their earliest actions upon taking office in 1979 was to increase the rate of Value Added Tax from 8% to 15%, which partly explains the subsequent rise in the rate of inflation. The Liberals sought to reduce inflation by a prices and incomes policy based on wide consultations but enforced by law, as well as by switching from taxing income to taxing wealth. They also suggested index-linked taxation on cigarettes and alcohol, a proposal with obvious merit to all concerned with better health. Labour's policy was to reduce inflation to 5% with the help of the TUC, to give more power to the Prices Commission, and to exert greater control over financial institutions, including more competition for the banks.

One could argue that of these three policies, the Liberals were the most radical, for with no business or trade union vote to worry about, they could tackle the problems with a straightforward prices policy (affecting firms) and incomes policy (affecting workers). The Conservative sympathy with laissez-faire ideas shows in their approach to public expenditure and their preference for taxing spending rather than relying on income tax. Labour's plans involved more central control of prices and the financial system.

Responses to these policies by the voter would vary, but given national agreement on the importance of encouraging growth and slowing the rate of inflation, the choice of what party to vote for is rarely based on calm appraisal of the alternatives offered, combined with an understanding of the political philosophy behind them. Rather, voting depends on habit and the gut reaction to the question: 'but what is best for ME?'

What is best for the majority is not necessarily the best for those most in need. Lower taxation is for many of the population a more attractive proposal than increased public spending. Socialists may, through their desire for social justice and a more equal society, vote in a more altruistic way. But it is of course a minority of the middle class who hold socialist views: voting in Britain is still very much on class lines; working-class allegiance to the Labour Party is still very strong. Of course, the declared policies of a political party in the election period are usually tempered by the reality of problems faced in office. In the 1979 budget the income taxes of both poor and rich were reduced. In the 1980 budget the abolition of the 25% tax rate on the lowest portion of incomes had an adverse effect on the low-paid, and the largest tax concessions went to those with an income of more than £27,750 per annum.

In health services policy, the Conservative Party favours higher charges, (eg. prescription charges went up to £1 per item at the end of 1980), as well as the encouragement of private medical care. The Labour Party seeks an eventual end to all charges and the phasing-out of private beds in NHS hospitals. The sympathy of the Conservatives to the private sector, and the antipathy of Labour Party members towards it, is a stark difference between the parties, and echoes the laissez-faire versus collectivist arguments already mentioned.

As explained in Chapter 1, local government's action is constrained by central government, yet central government needs local government to implement its policies. Conservative-controlled local councils may well disagree with a conservative government's policy (eg. the Local Government Act 1980). When central and local government institutions are controlled by different parties, the conflict generated can be very strong.

Education policy

The best example of this tension between central and local government is in educational policy. Since the 1950's, one of the biggest ideological disagreements between the parties has been over the comprehensive school. The Labour Party sees in the 11+ examination and the grammar school a concentration of resources on an elite, and a continuing reflection of the social class take-up of education. Children of middle-class parents are proportionately much more likely to pass the 11+, go to grammar schools, stay on after the minimum school-leaving age and go on to further and higher education. Labour policy is to promote comprehensive schools, catering for children of all abilities. The Conservatives see the comprehensive school as a threat to standards of education, and likely to diminish the achievement level of the brightest children, with adverse effects as they progress through the educational system.

In 1964, the Labour government was elected with a commitment to introduce comprehensive schools. They did not legislate. Instead they sent a Circular to local education authorities asking them to submit plans for introducing a system of comprehensive education. Some Conservative-controlled education authorities did so, albeit reluctantly. Labour education authorities went ahead, with varying degrees of enthusiasm and speed. But some Conservative councils delayed submitting their plans until 1970 by which time a new Conservative government was in power, which withdrew Labour's Circular. During the late 1960's, hostility to the then Labour government had been reflected in the growing number of educational authorities coming under Conservative control.

During the early 1970's, the Conservative government discouraged comprehensive schools, although the proportion of Labour-controlled education authorities increased as voters showed the government how unpopular it was becoming! The electorate delivered the same message to the Labour government of 1974–1979, with local elections showing an increasing swing to the Conservatives, and the Labour government being defeated in the 1979 general election. The Labour government of 1974, elected again with comprehensive education as a part of its policy, decided to legislate to ensure that local education authorities went over to comprehensive education in the government's lifetime. The Education Act 1976 compelled local authorities to reorganise secondary schooling on comprehensive lines, thus pleasing Labour local authorities, if displeasing Conservative ones. In fact some Conservative authorities, like the London Boroughs of Kingston and Richmond, managed to delay going comprehensive despite the Act – which was repealed when the Conservative government elected in 1979 took office, leaving areas like Richmond and Kingston free to run a selective system with no threat of government interference. The percentage of secondary school children in comprehensive schools rose from 35·9% in 1971, to 70% by 1976, and to nearly 74% by 1977.

A further example of the differences between the parties on education was made clear when the Conservative government announced in 1979 that they were introducing an 'assisted places' scheme. This meant that the bright children of parents unable to afford the full cost of fee-paying schools might be helped to attend one. The implication was that the comprehensive schools were failing their brightest children. The major problem of such 'creaming-off' is that schools with growing but small sixth forms could lose the one or two brightest pupils who might be a relatively large proportion of the abler children in the school, and the school might then be less able to cater for its remaining bright children! At a time when education expenditure by local authorities has had to be cut, and charges for such basic items as school meals are rising rapidly, the scheme's implementation is a clear indication of its ideological importance. The extent to which the hostility of the National Union of Teachers, as expressed at its 1980 Conference, will affect the scheme is unclear.

Both parties remain committed to more parental choice, and the Labour Party included reduced class sizes and an end to fee-paying independent schools in its 1979 manifesto. Public expenditure cuts fall particularly hard on education, although falling school rolls ease this slightly.

The dilemma of public expenditure cuts

Ironically, the public expenditure cuts are hitting hardest the local authority departments with the most rapidly rising demand – the social services departments. These departments are faced with rising expectations, rising numbers of the elderly and disabled, and more family stress as unemployment spreads and the proportion of one-parent families grows. The cut-backs in local authority spending can only make the life of the community nurse more difficult, as other community support services (eg. home helps, residential institutions) are reduced. In hospitals, the nurse may well find that the discharge of patients who need social care and support in their own homes will be delayed.

The extent to which Labour councils resist the cuts in public expenditure varies. It depends on the political mix within the Labour majority of each Labour-controlled council. Overall resistance to the cuts may mean very heavy rates rises for people living in the area. Radical Labour groups such as the councillors of the London

Borough of Lambeth showed active resistance to any public expenditure cuts. Whilst cutting with less enthusiasm than Conservative-controlled boroughs, other Labour councils bowed to the inevitable and began to cut back. Even without the actual cuts, rising inflation and reducing government help to local authorities means higher rates and a lower level of service provision.

The dilemma for the nurse is a stark one. She works face-to-face with those whose needs are not being met. Her own skills are likely to be used more extensively and so perhaps less effectively, and yet, as a ratepayer, and taxpayer she may welcome lower rates and reductions in income tax. One solution may be for a much more radical redistribution of wealth and income than even the Labour Party has yet been able to introduce. More likely is a shift towards higher charges and more direct payment by users, increasing the complexity of the operation of the welfare state for its most vulnerable users.

The 1979 Conservative government obviously hopes that the public expenditure cuts being made in the early 1980's will lead in the long run to increased growth, enabling increased spending on public services to be financed from the wealth generated from that growth.

This chapter has only been able to scratch the surface of the current political scene in relation to the provision of social services. It is hoped that readers will be helped to a better understanding of what is being decided in their own local area, and how such decisions are reached, as well as a better understanding of the national scene. Perhaps readers will be stimulated to take part in the debates now raging about some of these issues. In a democracy, such debates are healthy. Whichever side one takes in these debates, perhaps we should be grateful that we live in a society where the debate, whether at home, at work, or in the press, can take place without adverse effects on our family and professional lives. This is the reality behind the more theoretical discussion in Chapter 2 and the more thorough economic analysis of Chapters 4 and 5.

References

Beveridge W. (1942) *Social Insurance and Allied Services*. Cmd
        6404. London: HMSO

Calvocoressi P. (1978) *The British Experience 1945–75.*
    Harmondsworth, Middx.: Penguin
Moroney R. M. (1976) *The Family and the State: Considerations
    for Social Policy.* London: Longmans
Wilensky H. (1975) *The Welfare State and Equality.* University of
    California Press
Young M. & Wilmott P. (1973) *The Symmetrical Family: A Study
    of Work and Leisure in the London Region.* London:
    Routledge & Kegan Paul

Chapter 4

Paying for Services

Lesley Rimmer

It has been said that 'there is no such thing as a free lunch', and there is certainly no such thing as a *free* social service! Indeed, there are a number of different senses in which social services are *not free*. Firstly, we may actually be charged for consuming the service (although the charge may bear little relationship to the true cost). Secondly, we may pay for services through rates, taxes or national insurance contributions. Thirdly, we may use up other types of resources (time, energy) in obtaining supposedly free services: a good example of this is the time spent in doctors' waiting rooms or in out-patient departments at hospitals.

Apart from this, there is a fundamental *economic* sense in which social services are not free – any particular use of resources implies that they cannot at the same time be used for anything else. That is, there is an *opportunity cost* attached to any particular resource use. For example, the resources used to build a day centre for the elderly COULD have been used to build a nursery school, ie. the opportunity cost of the day centre IS the nursery school.

What is 'free' about some social services is that they are not priced at the 'point of consumption', that is, we do pay for them, but not *necessarily* at the time that we use them, and as individuals we do not necessarily pay the market price for them.

Public expenditure on the social services

Public expenditure on the five main social services (health, personal social services, education, housing and social security) in 1978–9 amounted to £38,046m, and total public expenditure over the same period amounted to £67,682m: thus, the social services accounted for 56% of total public spending (Social Trends 1979). Not only do the social services now absorb a very substantial proportion of public expenditure, but their rate of growth in expenditure terms has, until recently, been more rapid than that of public expenditure as a whole, and they have thus absorbed a *growing proportion* of public expenditure.

However, it is worth making some qualifications to these statements. Firstly, *total* expenditure on the social services comprises both public expenditure and private expenditure, for example, fees for private schooling and private medicine ought also to be included. Secondly, figures of public expenditure refer in the main to what is known as 'direct' expenditure, ie. actual expenditure from government revenues. However, an increasingly significant proportion of expenditure on a number of social services comes in the form of what the Americans call 'tax expenditures'. This refers to the revenue forgone by the goverrment when they 'give' tax allowances. One of the best known of these tax allowances, and one of the most costly, is the tax relief on mortgage interest. The interest which a person pays on a mortgage can be offset against his tax liability and in this way the Government has freed him from tax which he would otherwise have had to pay. In doing so it has given up revenue it would otherwise have received. This leaves the individual taxpayer, with a higher net income than he would otherwise receive whilst at the same time reducing government revenue.

These 'tax expenditures' have come to be seen by some as similar to the direct expenditures which they may complement or even replace. However, there is still some disagreement about whether this is a legitimate procedure. Whichever way one feels about this issue, it remains a fact that to ignore the 'opportunity cost' of tax allowances in certain fields is to vastly underestimate the extent of government 'effort' in that field. Let us follow the mortgage interest relief example a little further. In 1978–9 direct expenditure on housing was £4,923m: for the same year the 'opportunity cost' of the tax allowances on mortgage interest was £1,110m and thus, the total of government support to housing was £6,033m. (Inland Revenue 1979).

The issue of tax allowances becomes particularly important when we examine the distributional implications of alternative methods of financing the social services, since in essence tax relief is *regressive*, which means that those with higher incomes benefit most.

To return to our earlier statement of public expenditure, the third major qualification which needs to be made to these figures is the difference in the *nature* of the expenditure. A substantial part of the growth of public expenditure in recent years is accounted for by the growth of *transfer payments* such as pensions. These payments represent a redistribution of national resources from one part of the population to another (eg. from the working to the retired). They neither ADD to national resources nor do they SUBTRACT from them and, hence, are not included in the figures for Gross National Product (total income of UK residents from sources in the UK and abroad) or, as it is more commonly known, National Income. However, public expenditures, including transfers, are often related to the Gross National Product, or to the Gross Domestic Product (total value of goods and services produced in the UK), ie. described as a proportion of the total national wealth of Britain, and in this sense like is not really being compared with like. Indeed, some commentators go so far as to distinguish between the two different types of public expenditure, ie. *exhaustive* expenditure, which uses up real resources, and *transfers* which redistribute these resources, the best example of the latter being pensions, and of the former, expenditure on goods and services. Although this distinction is important in a number of contexts – debates about the growth of public expenditure being one – we shall not pursue it here. Suffice it to say that a substantial proportion of the increase in social services expenditure can be explained by the growth of transfer payments (particularly pensions, but expenditure on unemployment benefits is becoming more important), and by the rising cost of wages and salaries in the labour-intensive social services. The extent to which the post-war growth in public expenditure reflects the growth of these two categories is shown in Figure 4.1.

The NHS and the Personal Social Services

Perhaps more important than the level of expenditure on the social services is information on *how the money is spent.* Let us take the National Health Service and personal social services as an example. Table 4.1 shows the relationship of expenditure on the NHS to Britain's Gross Domestic Product (GDP) from 1949 onwards.

Two things are immediately apparent from this table. The first is that as a proportion of GDP, expenditure on the NHS has risen by

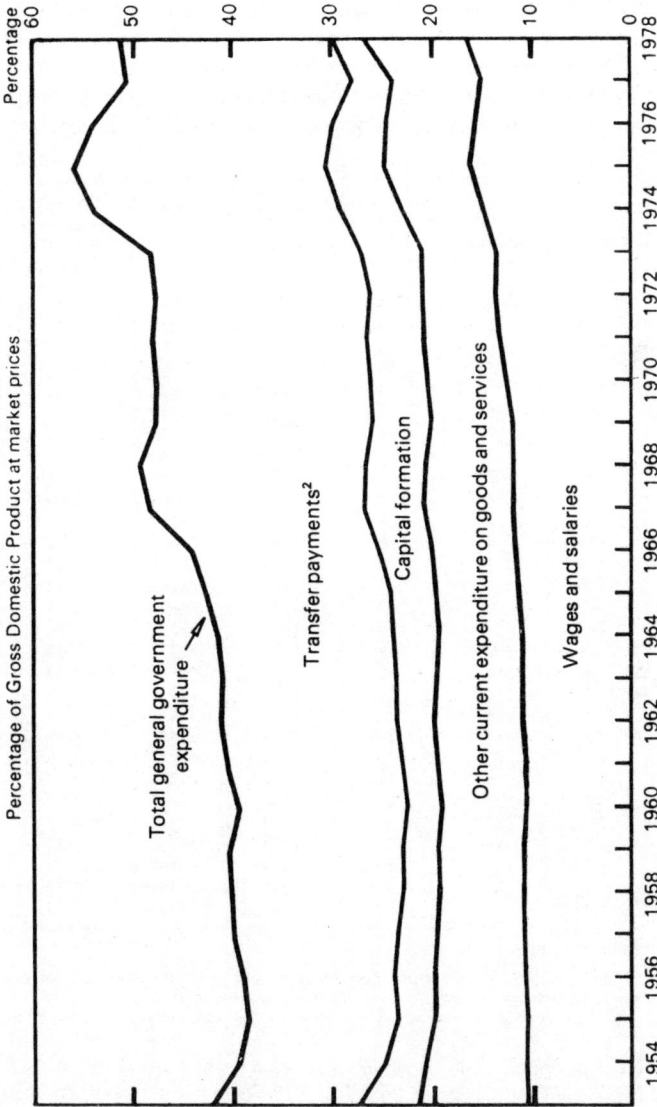

Fig 4.1 General government expenditure 1953 to 1978, by economic category (from *Social Trends 10*, 1979. Reproduced by permission of the Controller of Her Majesty's Stationery Office)

some 50% (and in real terms it has more than doubled). Secondly, by far the greater proportion of this expenditure relates to current or revenue expenditure; only a small proportion of total expenditure is on capital projects, such as hospital building. Indeed, some *three-quarters* of expenditure on the NHS goes on wages and salaries.

£million

Calendar year	NHS current	NHS capital	NHS other[2]	NHS total	GDP at factor cost	NHS total as percentage of GDP at factor cost
1949	414	15	4	433	10969	3.95
1950	458	16	4	478	11346	4.21
1951	476	17	6	499	12617	3.95
1952	476	15	6	497	13889	3.58
1953	500	16	5	521	14881	3.50
1954	515	18	4	537	15730	3.41
1955	555	20	4	579	16873	3.43
1956	609	20	4	633	18270	3.46
1957	655	26	4	685	19377	3.54
1958	694	29	5	728	20206	3.60
1959	750	34	4	788	21260	3.71
1960	819	37	5	861	22642	3.80
1961	879	44	5	928	24233	3.83
1962	909	55	7	971	25294	3.84
1963	968	60	7	1035	26894	3.85
1964	1047	76	7	1130	29255	3.86
1965	1176	91	8	1275	31237	4.08
1966	1290	102	9	1401	33139	4.23
1967[1]	1423	125	10	1558	34925	4.46
1968	1540	143	10	1693	37411	4.53
1969	1626	137	10	1773	39450	4.49
1970	1860	151	13	2024	43445	4.66
1971	2104	181	14	2299	49264	4.67
1972	2413	223	14	2650	54963	4.82
1973	2706	277	30	3013	63946	4.71
1974	3622	296	16	3934	73722	5.34
1975	4903	366	30	5299	92507	5.73
1976	5788	425	23	6236	109499	5.70
1977	6477	393	27	6897	123353	5.59

Source: health departments' statistics.

Notes: [1] Up to 1966 NHS current expenditure includes an imputed rent element; from 1967 this is replaced by a charge for non-trading capital consumption.
[2] Includes current grants to the personal sector and abroad and capital grants to the personal sector and to companies.

Table 4.1 NHS expenditure and Gross Domestic Product: UK 1949 to 1977 (from *Report of the Royal Commission on the NHS* 1979. Reproduced by permission of the Controller of Her Majesty's Stationery Office)

Table 4.2 examines the programmes which make up the current expenditure on the NHS and the personal social services. It is easy to see that expenditure on the hospital services dominates this table. Equally obvious are the relatively small amounts spent specifically on services for the mentally handicapped and mentally ill, despite the fact that mental illness accounts for over 40% of occupied hospital beds.

Paying for the social services

The National Health Service obtains most of its funds directly from the Exchequer. In 1978–9, 88% of NHS finance came from general taxation, 9·5% from the NHS part of national insurance contributions and 2% from prescription and other charges. It is the intention of the Conservative government elected in 1979 to raise the proportion of revenue obtained from charges, and, indeed, prescription charges were significantly increased in the 1980 Budget. Charges to NHS patients – excluding private patients – currently yield around £125m per annum, compared with an expenditure on the NHS in 1978–9 of £8,100m and therefore represents only 2·0% of NHS costs (Royal Commission on the NHS 1979). Half of this revenue comes from dental charges and a quarter each from charges for prescriptions and ophthalmic services.

The personal social services are financed to varying degrees from fees and charges. For residential care of the elderly, fees and charges represent some 30% of expenditure on that service and some 75% of all local authority revenue from fees and charges (Judge 1978). In contrast, charges for the residential care of children represent only 1·1% of expenditure on that service, and 1·4% of total revenue from charges.

We now turn to education, where we find some 88% of all education spending is undertaken by local education authorities, who obtain about half of their total revenue direct from the government in the form of a general grant – the Rate Support Grant – as discussed in Chapter 2, and specific grants. In addition, they obtain nearly one third of their revenue from the local rates. Local education authorities are responsible for the provision of primary, secondary and further education. They also bear prime responsibility for financing the public sector of higher education – the

Source: health departments' statistics. £million 1978 Public expenditure survey prices

		1975/76	1976/77	Provisional 1977/78
GRAND TOTAL		5989.2	6074.2	6213.1
PRIMARY CARE	Total	1202.9	1252.0	1259.8
Family Practitioner Services		1116.0	1169.1	1175.0
Prevention		13.9	15.6	15.1
Family Planning		13.0	12.9	12.7
Other Community Health		60.0	54.4	57.0
GENERAL & ACUTE HOSPITAL AND MATERNITY SERVICES	Total	2319.5	2334.0	2399.1
Acute IP and OP		1810.5	1800.2	1853.0
Ambulances		112.0	111.5	115.2
Other Hospital		164.8	190.5	197.1
Obstetric IP and OP		203.9	204.4	206.0
Midwives		28.3	27.4	27.8
SERVICES MAINLY FOR ELDERLY AND PHYSICALLY HANDICAPPED	Total	789.3	801.3	820.3
Geriatric IP and OP[1]		282.9	286.0	292.8
Non-Psychiatric DP		13.3	17.1	18.6
District Nursing		84.9	91.7	92.9
Chiropody		13.6	12.2	12.7
Residential Care		180.6	182.3	183.4
Home Help		112.1	113.2	115.8
Meals		16.2	16.3	16.4
Day Care		21.4	23.5	26.2
Aids, Adaptations, Phones etc.		13.6	12.6	12.7
Services for the Disabled		50.7	46.4	44.1
SERVICES FOR MENTALLY HANDICAPPED	Total	250.6	251.9	263.0
Mental Handicap IP and OP		199.5	195.8	202.2
Residential Care		20.3	23.4	26.5
Day Care		30.8	32.7	34.3
SERVICES FOR MENTALLY ILL	Total	455.7	446.4	464.7
Mental Illness IP and OP		417.8	406.3	420.6
Psychiatric DP		16.5	17.7	20.4
Residential Care		4.6	5.1	5.8
Day Care		3.6	4.0	4.3
Special Hospital		13.2	13.3	13.6
SERVICES MAINLY FOR CHILDREN	Total	329.7	340.5	351.0
Health Visiting		49.1	49.0	52.0
School Health		57.0	54.9	57.8
Welfare Food		18.3	20.1	20.4
Residential Care		148.7	153.8	153.7
Boarding Out		17.7	20.6	23.4
Day Nurseries		33.4	36.4	36.7
Intermediate Treatment		1.0	1.1	2.0
Central Grants and YTCs		4.5	4.6	5.0
OTHER SERVICES	Total	641.5	648.1	655.2
Social Work		111.6	114.8	119.1
Other Local Authority Services		29.1	26.9	29.1
Hospital and Community Health Admin.		214.5	221.2	219.8
Local Authority Administration		140.5	141.4	143.4
Centrally Financed Services		145.8	143.8	143.8

Notes [1] Includes units for younger disabled.

[2] Abbreviations: DP, IP, OP, YTCs - Day patients, In-patients, Out-patients, Youth Treatment Centres

[3] A fuller explanation of the methodology of the Programme Budget from which these figures are devised can be found in Annex 2 of the DHSS Consultative Document "Priorities for Health and Personal Social Services in England", published by HMSO in 1976, and also in Appendix VI of the follow-up document, "The Way Forward", published in September 1977.

Table 4.2 NHS and PSS current expenditure by Programme: England 1975/76 to 1977/78 (from *Report of the Royal Commission on the NHS* 1979. Reproduced by permission of the Controller of Her Majesty's Stationery Office)

Polytechnics — although they obtain resources from the Local Authorities Financial Pool. The universities obtain most of their funds from central government via the University Grants Committee and, in addition, obtain funds from fees, rents and investments.

Turning to housing, nearly 55% of the housing stock is owner-occupied and this highlights the importance of tax relief, as discussed earlier in this chapter, to the overall financing of housing. Private expenditure, therefore, represents a much more substantial proportion of spending on housing than it does on other social services.

Public expenditure on housing includes the cost of rent rebates and allowances to council and private tenants, and the much larger sums involved in building and maintaining local authority housing. In 1977–8 the average local authority tenant 'received' £290 per annum in public funds, the average person with a mortgage £199 and the private tenant only £39 per annum (Social Trends 1978). Housing provisions are discussed in Chapter 8.

With regard to social security, as indicated earlier in this chapter, social security benefits are transfer payments. Although it is popularly believed that the contributory nature of the social security system means that an individual pays for his or her own pension (that is, a transfer occurs over an individual's own lifetime), the truth is that *today's pensioners* have their pensions financed by the contributions of *today's working population*. That is, the system works on a pay-as-you-go basis. However, it is in the interest of the policymakers to encourage the contributory myth, since they argue that national insurance contributions are a more 'popular' form of taxation than income tax.

National insurance benefits are based on the principle of 'contingency redistribution', which means there is a redistribution from the well to the sick; the employed to the unemployed and so on. Supplementary Benefit entitlement is based on a means test. It is, therefore, difficult to determine the overall distributive impact of these benefits since the redistribution of income is not their primary objective. The major source of finance for National Insurance benefits is contributions, some 82%, with a small supplement from the Consolidated Fund (general tax revenue), amounting to about 15%. In contrast, Supplementary Benefits are ALL financed from general tax revenue, with nothing from contributions.

Public expenditure cuts

Public expenditure on the health and social services rose sharply in the 1960's and early 1970's but in recent years the level of public expenditure has been reduced from previously announced expenditure plans. The 1979 Conservative government went further, and plans a reduction in the actual level of public expenditure in 1980–81, compared to the level in 1979–80. Overall, this reduction is from £71,776m to £70,729m. In the major social services, the reduction is from £43,204m to £42,807m.

The implications of the current round of public expenditure cuts are complex, and there is no room in a book of this length to explore these issues in depth. The impact of these cuts is, no doubt, becoming increasingly clear to those working in the NHS, and readers can make their own judgement on the effects of the cuts on the services they are providing to patients.

The distribution of the social services

It is often argued that the social services are distributed on the basis of 'need'. However, in practice, degrees of need prove very difficult to determine (Bradshaw 1972). The social services depend heavily on professional workers, who, as they exercise professional discretion, determine the allocation of resources between different clients. They choose patients, students and tenants ... and thus indirectly allocate resources between these different clients, and so between regions, specialisms, schools, and so on.

However, distribution of resources on this basis may not accord with concepts of 'territorial justice', ie. the distribution of services between geographical areas, nor with concepts like equity. In particular, the regional and geographical imbalance in the provision of health services has been the subject of a study by the Resource Allocation Working Party (DHSS 1976) which is discussed in Chapter 6. Apart from the centralised re-allocation of resources as suggested by this Working Party, an alternative method of changing the allocation of resources between individuals, or groups, is to introduce user charges. The debate about charges is wider than simply the distributional one, however, and it has become a central issue in the debate about the financing of health services.

Charges in the social services

What is the case for user charges? People who advocate the increased use of charges in the health and social services do so on a
number of different grounds, and the history of charges for these services provides many examples of changing emphasis and reasons for
charges (Parker 1976).

In part, the argument about charges is an aspect of the wider
debate about the role of the *market* as opposed to *public provision*
discussed in the first chapters of this book. It is important to distinguish between the various levels at which the case can be argued.
Some commentators would prefer the provision of what are now the
social services on a totally private basis: the production of services
would be on a private, normally profit-making, basis, and the distribution or allocation of the services would be through charges, ie.
based on the ability to pay, just as for the supply of apples or other
goods. An example would be a private hospital whose patients paid
the full-cost fees for the services they received. This is a somewhat
extreme example, and there are many less extreme versions. For
example, the patients might not be required to pay fees which
covered the full cost of the services they consumed as individuals,
but some average cost which would, when taken as a whole, cover
the total running costs of the hospital. Similarly, we need not assume
that the patients would pay the total costs of their treatment out of
current income or savings, since private insurance schemes could be
used to pool the risks between members of the schemes.

Other advocates of charges are concerned with less radical
changes. Within a framework of publicly-provided services they
propound charging the consumer as a way of minimising the 'waste'
which they believe is caused by the irresponsible use of free services.
Such proposals are often linked to a more generous scheme of
exemptions from charges to protect vulnerable or needy groups.
Indeed, the elderly, children and the mentally and physically handicapped absorb some 60% of NHS expenditure but are unlikely to be
appropriate groups on which to levy increased charges.

It is thus important to recognise that ideas about the use of
charges form only one part of the wider continuum of ideas which
runs from a totally private system at one pole, to a free, publicly-
provided service at the other, with allocation of resources on the

basis of need. It is also important to distinguish whether one is primarily concerned to introduce these principles into the *production* of services as well as, or in contrast to, the *distribution* of services. In the former case, the principal logic is that of increasing the 'efficiency' of production both in terms of its responsiveness to consumer preferences, and in terms of creating a consciousness of the real resource costs of services through the use of pricing. In the latter case, the *distribution* of services on the basis of market principles, is primarily related to concern with the level of consumption of free services and the raising of additional revenue. Indeed, concern with 'abuse', waste and the raising of additional funds are central themes in the charges debate.

At first sight the case for charges is intuitively appealing: if charges for services are introduced, it is argued, people will think twice about whether they really need the services. There is the suspicion that if the services are 'free' people will consume more than they otherwise would, and that to perpetuate free services is to invite both abuse and waste (Harris & Seldon 1979). On closer inspection, however, the argument has less force. Firstly, in the NHS in particular, but also within other areas of social service provision, the consumer does *not* have independent access to services. Access is decided by the professionals: general practitioners, consultants, and so on. Thus, it is not open to us to arrive at a local hospital and demand that an appendix be removed – unless we arrive as an emergency case, we will have had to consult our family doctor, be referred to a consultant and have had our case for admission vetted by these two professionals. At this level, certainly, it would be difficult for the patient to abuse the use of health services without the collusion of members of the medical profession! As the Royal Commission on the NHS (1979) pointed out, 'It follows that there can be little abuse of hospital resources by patients, and that if incentives and disincentives are to have a major effect on the use of hospital resources then they must be offered to doctors and not to patients'.

Secondly, few of us would willingly subject ourselves to unnecessary medical procedures.

Thirdly, to restrict access to services in the short run may be costly in the longer term. Early diagnosis is important for efficient treatment of a number of diseases, and to delay until a critical condition is reached is often very costly: to the patient as well as to the health service!

It is important to specify *where* a charge is to fall. Let us explore two examples: prescription charges, and charges for visits to the general practitioner (GP). If, having visited the GP and obtained a prescription, the charge deters us from having it filled, will waste have been decreased or increased? In the short run, the drugs bill will be lower than it otherwise would have been, but on the other hand, if the prescription was an important part of the treatment obtained from the visit to the GP, then the visit itself has in some senses been wasted. Concern with the rising cost of pharmaceuticals is now being reflected in a programme of re-education of patients so that they do not expect a prescription every time they visit the doctor, and in some faltering, and vigorously contested, attempts to constrain the prescribing habits of GPs within certain limits (Abel-Smith 1976). Charges for visits to the GP have been regularly suggested as a way both of raising additional revenue and reducing his workload.

Although, as has been shown, charges currently raise a very small proportion of revenue in the NHS, the Royal Commission (1979) produced estimates, based on the 1975–76 financial year, of the effect of prescription charges of 50p per item, an 'hotel' charge for in-patients of £20 per week, an accident and emergency visit fee of £5, and £2 for consulting one's GP. With unchanged dental and ophthalmic service charges, and taking account both of administrative costs of collecting the charges and of reductions in the use of services, they estimated the new charges could generate some £423m of additional revenue – only 8·0% of NHS expenditure in 1975–6.

These calculations did not incline the Royal Commission to recommend charges of this sort. With regard to charges for visits to GPs, the Commission ask, 'would the extra administrative costs and inconveniences of charges be compensated for by keeping away from GPs those who demand their services frivolously? We doubt it, and we would be uneasy that it could well discourage patients from seeking help when they really needed it'. Indeed, on balance, they concluded '. . . we feel that, particularly with the irrational structure of charges we now have, there is a good case for their gradual but complete extinction, and we so recommend'.

So far, charges which affect the *distribution* of services have been discussed. There have also been calls for some form of pricing of the *production* of services, so that both practitioners and patients understand the true cost of the resources being consumed, and can make better decisions about the way resources are used. Examples of such pricing include making clear the alternative cost of therapies and showing the implications of different policies on length of hospital stay. This is particularly important in a period of financial stringency when the public's expectations about the growth in available resources is unlikely to be met.

As the Regional Administrators of RHAs (England) in their evidence to the Royal Commission on the NHS said: 'The NHS has become accustomed throughout the 25 years preceding the re-organisation to the prospect of continual growth in the financial resources available to it. Though agreeable, the result has been to allow slack management, with no incentive to examine obsolete patterns of spending, or to develop a coherent plan for the future.'

We have shown that the resources available to the NHS have doubled in real terms since 1949 (see Table 4.1), yet in evidence to the Royal Commission the British Medical Association argued '... for some years now the money allocated by the government for the Service has been quite inadequate to meet the demands made upon it by the public', and one medical witness went so far as to say that '... we can easily spend the whole of the gross national product'! It is however unlikely that the resources available to the NHS will increase as rapidly as before and, therefore, it is especially important to plan the efficient utilisation of available resources. There is a need for long-term planning, both for medical and other manpower and for the best use of capital programmes.

The major social services have not been insulated from the public expenditure cuts, which are often imposed at short notice. One of the saddest aspects of this is that cuts have had to be made quickly and in an arbitrary fashion, which can itself lead to the *inefficient* use of resources. Again, readers may have come across examples of this from their personal experience within the health and social services.

Who benefits from the social services?

Who pays and who benefits from the social services? Such seemingly simple questions are deceptive because they are particularly difficult to answer. We have seen that taxation in various forms provides most of the finance for the social services, and therefore one might think that the simple answer 'the taxpayer pays' would be sufficient. However, it is important to realise that revenue raised from taxation is not raised equally from every individual. It is generally accepted that the tax taken by the government in the form of direct taxes (primarily taxes on income) takes a similar proportion of income from all income groups, and so is only mildly progressive. The evidence on the incidence of indirect taxes (ie. taxes on expenditure) is even less clear.

If the question 'who pays for the social services?' is difficult to answer, then the question 'who benefits?' is even more so. The difficulty is partly theoretical and partly methodological. To the question 'who benefits from the education services?' there are at least three answers: children, teachers and society. To some extent, education is what is known as a *public good*, that is, its benefits are spread throughout the population and not limited to the individuals undergoing that education, but it is also true that education is a *private good*, the benefit of which can be confined primarily to the individual. For example, the benefit of a university education can be seen in the individual's lifetime earnings which are usually higher than the earnings of someone who left school at 16. On this basis children benefit as individuals, and society as a whole benefits from having an educated population. But it can also be argued that the main beneficiaries of the education service are the providers of that service – teachers, administrators, etc., whose employment is generated and sustained by the service. Thus, it is possible to consider the 'benefit' of a service on a number of different bases.

Methodologically, the question of determining the distribution of benefits is also difficult. With a number of the social services the benefit depends on the use made of the services. Social scientists have analysed according to social class, the use made of the health service, and it has been shown that the higher social classes – professionals, employers and managers, together with their families – obtain up to 40% more health service expenditure for every person reporting an illness than the semi-skilled and unskilled manual workers (Le Grand 1978; DHSS 1980). This same pattern has also been shown in education (Glennerster 1975).

This type of analysis highlights the question of access to the social services. In so far as access is mediated by professionals, and different social groups respond differently to professional workers, then it seems likely that the disproportionate utilisation of services by professional groups will persist.

Nurses, as one of these professional groups, have an important role to play in *widening* access to services, ie. making it easier for the more inarticulate members of society to make their needs known. The importance of this should become clearer as readers turn to Chapter 6, in which the NHS is examined in more detail.

References

Abel-Smith B. (1976) *Value for Money in the Health Services*. London: Heinemann

Bradshaw J. (1972) A taxonomy of social need. In McLachlan G. (ed) *Problems and Progress in Medical Care, 7th Series*. Oxford University Press

Central Statistical Office (1978) *Social Trends 9*. London: HMSO

Central Statistical Office (1979) *Social Trends 10*. London: HMSO

DHSS (1976) *Sharing Resources for Health in England: Report of the Resource Allocation Working Party*. London: HMSO

DHSS (1980) *Inequalities in Health: Report of a Research Working Group*. London: HMSO

Glennerster H. (1973) Education and inequality. In Bosanquet N. & Townsend P. (eds) *Labour and Inequality*. London: Fabian Society

Glennerster H. (1975) *Social Service Budgets and Social Policy*. London: Allen & Unwin

Harris R. & Seldon A. (1979) *Over-ruled on Welfare*. London: Institute of Economic Affairs

Inland Revenue (1979) *Inland Revenue Statistics*. London: HMSO

Judge K. (1978) *Rationing Social Services*. London: Heinemann

Le Grand J. (1978) Who benefits from public expenditure? *New Society*, 21 Sept.

Parker R. A. (1976) Charging for the social services. *Journal of Social Policy*, 5(4)

Royal Commission on the National Health Service (Chairman: Sir Alec Merrison) (1979) *Report*. Cmnd 7615. London: HMSO

Chapter 5

Did Poverty Die when the Welfare State was Born?

Lesley Rimmer

The modern welfare state can be said to be the child of the post-Second World War era of reconstruction, although its antecedents go back much further, and as we saw in Chapter 2 it is the framework provided by the Beveridge Report (1942) that is central to its development.

Beveridge's objective was to eliminate *want* – the most important of his five 'giant' evils. His plan encompassed a comprehensive scheme of social insurance which was to cover all the main causes of interruption of earnings, linked to a plan for full employment, a free NHS, and a system of universal family allowances.

The 'social insurance' part of the plan had two parts: an *insurance* scheme in which benefits were to be earned by contributions, and an *assistance* scheme with non-contributory but means-tested benefits, which would provide the 'safety net' of the system. The role of the assistance provisions was to become a *residual* one once the coverage of the insurance scheme was complete. This meant that it would help those with too few contributions to qualify for social insurance benefits and would then be used as a last resort for those not fully covered for other reasons, eg. disability. Since it would take time for the insurance scheme to be complete – twenty years or more in the case of pensions – it is evident that poverty would not be eliminated overnight.

An outline of the major benefits available is given at the end of this chapter, although it should be noted that legislation relating to social security changes and to changes in tax allowances are frequent.

Thirty years on, however, it is obvious that poverty has still not been eliminated – indeed, one estimate puts the proportion of families living below the poverty level as high as 29% (Layard *et al.* 1978). Why is this? A large part of the explanation lies in the way in which we define poverty – a matter about which there is a continuing debate.

Defining poverty

The pioneering attempts to define poverty were those of Booth (1890) and Rowntree (1901), whose work in investigating the causes of poverty was important, as we saw in Chapter 2, in helping society to see that poverty was not necessarily an individual's fault. Rowntree, in his study of York in 1899, attempted to cost diet and clothing at a level which would be adequate merely to maintain physical efficiency. Important to the concept, and to people's view of the poor, was the distinction which he made between primary and secondary poverty. Primary poverty existed where income was inadequate to provide a basic level of subsistence, whereas secondary poverty existed if, despite having enough money, the family failed to spend its income on the necessities to maintain life and health.

Rowntree and others were primarily concerned with an *absolute* view of poverty – that is a level which could be defined in terms of nutritional intake sufficient for subsistence. However, it is obvious that an absolute standard in a time of change in the living standards of the majority of the population is of limited usefulness.

The alternative view of poverty is that it is *relative* to the time and society under consideration: this has the obvious merit of being closer to a generally accepted view of poverty. This concept defines people as poor if they have insufficient income to participate normally in the society in which they live – to be able to eat out occasionally, buy new clothes, keep warm in winter, and so on. It is also important to realise that what constitutes poverty in one country may be relative affluence in another – poverty in India is obviously far worse in absolute terms than that found in Britain. At the same time a relative view of poverty has one important limitation: if the poorest tenth of the population is viewed as being in poverty, then in one sense the poor are always with us!

An alternative way, which has been frequently used in modern studies of poverty, is to take a poverty line based on the levels of living 'guaranteed' by the Supplementary Benefits scheme, which is the modern equivalent of the National Assistance scheme set up by Beveridge. Although this approach can be criticised (for example, on the basis of the relative needs implied between adults and children in the scale rates payable), it has a number of advantages. Firstly, the Supplementary Benefits scheme is in effect the State's own 'poverty line' – the line below which, in prescribed circumstances, the State will supplement an individual's income. The Supplementary Benefit (SB) levels are also the bases of the 'prescribed levels' in the Family Income Supplement (FIS) scheme, which is a parallel means-tested benefit for low-wage working families with children. Secondly, the levels of SB payments are uprated periodically to take account of changes in the cost of living.

It is useful therefore to use the SB levels to define the numbers in poverty. However, it is not sufficient to take the SB levels as they stand. There are a number of *different* poverty lines, depending on the composition of the family in question, whether there are any 'exceptional' circumstances such as a medical need for a diet requiring additional foods, and whether the beneficiaries are long-term, like the elderly, or short-term, like the unemployed who after one year lose their entitlement to unemployment benefit.

In addition, those eligible for Supplementary Benefits have their rent paid (if it is thought to be reasonable) and are eligible for rates rebates, as well as mortgage interest in the case of owner-occupiers. Thus, some adjustment needs to be made for housing costs.

In the study by Layard *et al.* (1978), income (after housing costs have been taken into account) is used, and is related to the long-term SB entitlement of households of given composition. On this basis they estimate that in 1975 $4\frac{1}{2}$ million people lived on annual incomes at or below the long-term SB level. Another $4\frac{1}{2}$ million were below an income level of 120% of SB, and a further 5 million were below 140% of this level: that is, were very near poverty. These different levels obviously represent different degrees of poverty, but if we take the 140% cut-off point, then some 14 million people or 26% of the population live below this level (29% of all families).

The poor defined

Who are the poor? Which groups are most likely to be in poverty? It is important to make a distinction between the risk of poverty for any particular group, that is the *proportion* of that group who are living in poverty, and the *accountability* of that group – that is, what proportion of all those who are poor is represented by the group. It is possible, therefore, to have family types which have a high risk of poverty (ie. a high *proportion* of that group are poor) but which have a low accountability (ie. family of that type represent only a *small* proportion of those who are in poverty). A good example of this type of family is the single-parent family, which exhibits high risk but low accountability.

One very useful way of highlighting these factors is to use the 'poverty tree' approach of the Layard *et al.* (1978) study which is reproduced as Figures 5.1 & 5.2.

Figure 5.1 shows the percentage of families in each category which have household incomes below 140% of SB. It shows therefore the types of families in which the risk of poverty is higher than for all families, and those where it is lower. For all families, the risk of poverty is 29%, for elderly people (men over 65, women over 60), the risk is 64% – twice the 'normal' risk! In contrast, for non-elderly couples the risk is only 14% (half 'normal' risk), and for single people it is 18%.

This poverty tree approach also enables us to compare the *relative* risk of groups with different attributes. For example, among elderly people not working, the risk of poverty is 69%, compared to a risk of 28% when they are able to continue working. Similarly, working single-parent families have a 37% risk, compared to a risk of 87% for non-working single parents, who are usually dependent on SB, widow's benefit or maintenance from ex-husbands.

The relative risk of poverty in various groups is obviously important to policy makers, but perhaps more important is the *composition* of poverty – that is, who the poor are. In this case, if priority is to be given to reducing poverty it is the groups which account for the highest *proportion* of those in poverty on whom attention should focus.

Figure 5.2 shows how the poor population is made up, and therefore, how various groups account for different proportions of those in poverty. The elderly account for 57% of the poor (made up of 54% non-working elderly and 3% working elderly). Single parents account for 6% of the poor, 4% not being in employment, and 2% in employment. In fact, compared with all the other family types, including single people, single parents form the smallest group in poverty.

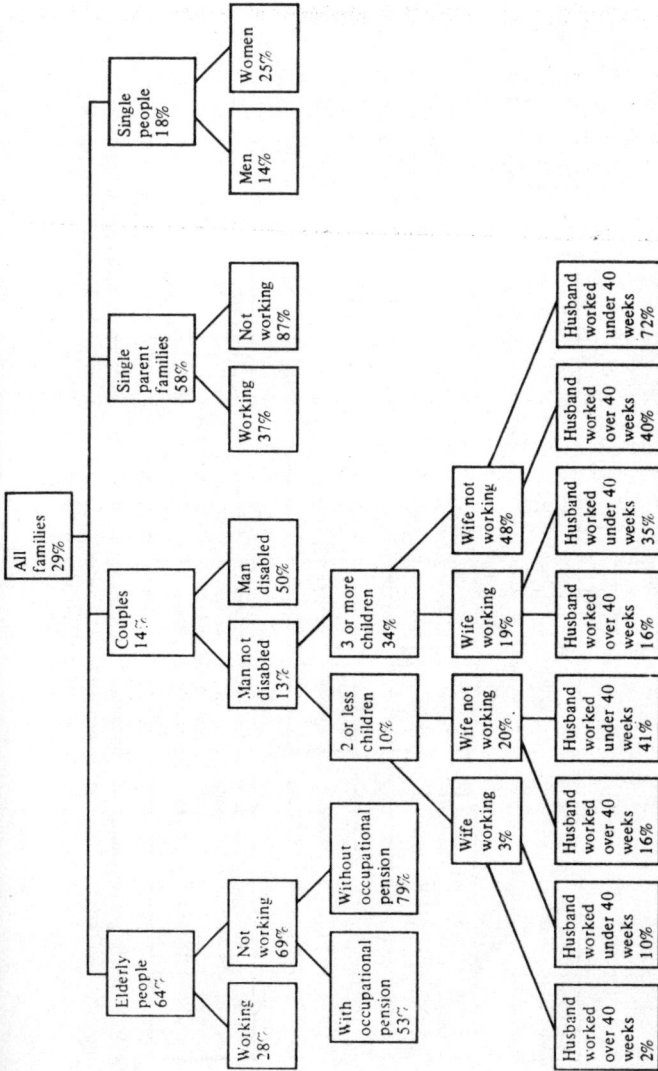

Note: The number given in each box gives the percentage of the group of families defined by the corresponding 'branch' of the tree who have a household income of below 140 per cent of SB.

Fig 5.1 Percentages of families in each category having household income below 140% of SB (from *Royal Commission on the Distribution of Income and Wealth, Background Paper No. 5* 1978. Reproduced by permission of the Controller of Her Majesty's Stationery Office)

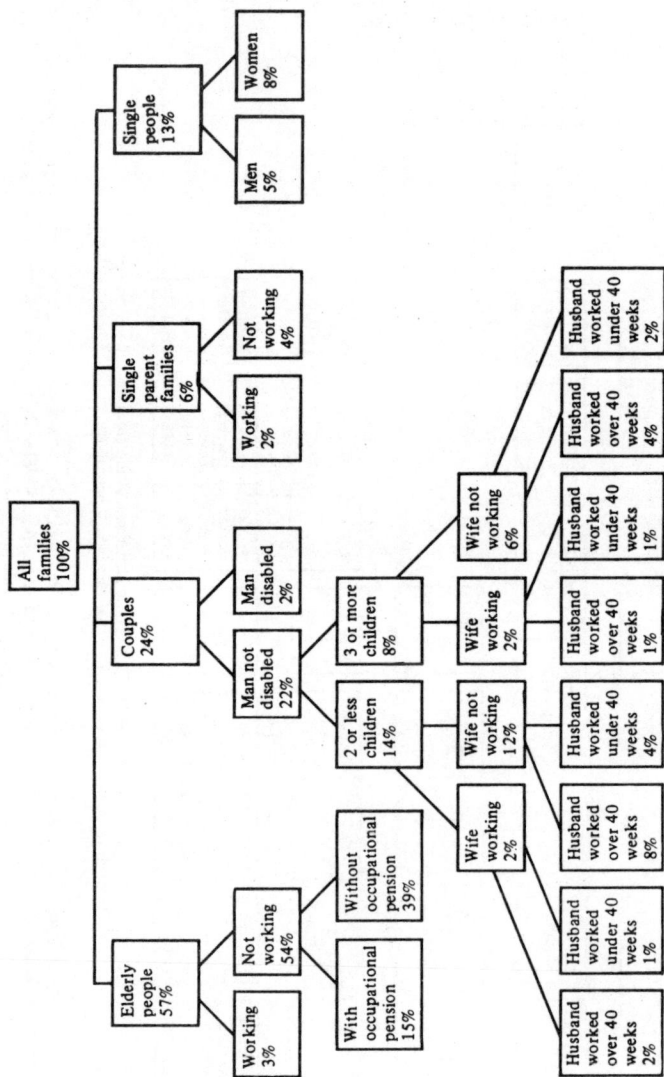

Fig 5.2 Percentages of families with household incomes below 140% of SB which are in each type of family (from *Royal Commission on the Distribution of Income and Wealth, Background Paper No. 5* 1978. Reproduced by permission of the Controller of Her Majesty's Stationery Office)

The groups most at risk of poverty

What are the implications of this approach to poverty? In terms of an efficient anti-poverty strategy, it means that effort should be concentrated on those groups which exhibit both high risk and high accountability. The group which fits this description precisely is the elderly, and in particular, the non-working elderly without occupational pensions.

What about other groups? Single-parent families with a non-working head have the *highest risk of poverty* (87%) of all the groups identified, but this group *accounts for only 4% of the poor*. Perhaps this fact is one explanation of the inactivity which followed publication of the comprehensive report on the financial and social situation of one parent families, The Finer Report (1974).

It is important to stress two points about this analysis. Firstly, that the number of people in poverty is critically dependent on where the poverty line is drawn and, secondly, that this also affects the composition of the poor. Indeed, the pioneering study which awoke concern about poverty in Britain in the 1960's was called *The Poor and the Poorest* (Abel-Smith & Townsend 1965).

Let us next consider the composition of poverty at various degrees of poverty. Of those with household income below 100% of SB (that is, the very poorest), 48% are elderly, with a disproportionate number of single women; 28% are couples with children, and 15% are single parents. In the groups with income between 100%–120% of SB, pensioners constitute 39%, but two-parent families constitute 43% of the total with single parents having fallen to 8%. Similarly, as we move to 120–140% of SB, the proportion of pensioners falls dramatically to 24%, and single parents to 4%, while two-parent couples with children increase to 56%. Therefore we can see that the two groups which are disproportionately represented among the *poorest* are the elderly and the single-parent families.

But surely, it could be argued that there is something paradoxical in defining the number in poverty on the basis of the levels of living guaranteed by the SB scheme? This scheme, after all, is meant to guarantee incomes at least equal to 100% of SB entitlement – how is it, then, that anyone falls *below* this level?

To understand the answer to this question it is necessary to describe briefly the structure of the social security system. The scheme is not described here in detail, nor are benefit amounts given, as they change frequently. Instead, readers are advised to obtain a comprehensive booklet entitled *Family Benefits* (reference FB1) from their local social security office. This booklet is published to assist those in the caring professions who may wish to help clients or patients, and as such, social workers and nurses may obtain a copy. A summary of the benefits available will be found at the end of this chapter.

The social security system

The basic structure of the present social security system is still based on the recommendations of the Beveridge Report. As we have noted, Beveridge's proposals for reform rested on three assumptions: that poverty related to family size would be eliminated by a system of family allowances, that positive government actions would prevent mass unemployment, and that there would be a freely-available comprehensive health service. His insurance scheme was based on the payment of a flat-rate benefit for all contingencies causing a loss of earnings. There were to be additions to benefit for dependants, and the level of benefit was to provide a subsistence level of income. The scheme was to be comprehensive in coverage, with people insured either on the basis of their own contributions, or, in the case of married women, on the basis of their husbands' contributions.

Given the contributory nature of the scheme it was felt to be inappropriate to link payment of benefit to a test of means or needs and consequently insurance benefits are paid irrespective of other income (although no more than one benefit is normally payable at any one time).

Despite the fact that the scheme was intended to be comprehensive, Beveridge recognised that there would always be some individuals who would fail to meet the contribution conditions (ie. the requirement to have paid a certain number of contributions in the years preceding a claim). This would exclude categories such as the young person who has only recently begun to work and the person who is too disabled to find a job. He therefore linked the *insurance* scheme to an *assistance* scheme of benefits. The assistance scheme was also designed for those who were exempted from national insurance contributions on the basis of insufficient income, and for those whose needs were greater. This assistance scheme is now known as Supplementary Benefits (SB).

It was evident that until the insurance scheme reached maturity, reliance on the assistance benefits, which would be means-tested, would persist, but it was believed that this would decline as the coverage of the insurance scheme system increased.

A third branch of the scheme was the Industrial Injuries provisions, originally introduced by the Workmen's Compensation Act 1897. Provision both for injury at work and for industrially-induced diseases was to be financed from contributions from employers, employees, and a levy on the more dangerous industries. Benefits in this scheme were to be related to loss of earning power.

Although most of the recommendations of the Beveridge Report were implemented in the immediate post-war period, there were some important limitations. In 1944 the Government accepted responsibility for maintaining a high and stable level of employment, Family Allowances (now changed in form to become Child Benefit), were introduced in 1946, and the NHS was established in 1948. The National Insurance and Industrial Injuries Acts, which came into force in 1948, contained most of the recommendations for social security itself. However, the industrial injuries scheme was financed on the same basis as that for national insurance.

The main structure of the scheme still exists today, although the rates of all benefits and allowances have been revised a number of times and are now (except for Child Benefit) uprated *annually*. Under the Social Security Pensions Act 1975 the regulations required the uprating of long-term benefits in line with either earnings or prices (current government proposals will change this to uprating on the basis of prices only). However, inadequacies in the scheme soon became apparent and its structure began to change, albeit slowly.

Changes in the social security system   The principle of flat-rate benefits in return for flat-rate contributions was limited in terms of contribution level by the contributions which the lowest earners in the scheme could be expected to meet. Even the lowest flat-rate contribution was a relatively high proportion of income for the low-paid, if negligible for the better-off. This also meant that the flat-rate benefit represented a substantial drop in income, especially on retirement, for higher income earners. A partial solution to this dilemma was afforded by the National Insurance Act 1959 which introduced a graduated (earnings-related) pension system from 1961. Under these arrangements, contributions for retirement pensions were partially related to earnings, so that higher earners contributed more, to be repaid by a higher eventual pension. The same principle of graduated contributions and benefits was extended in October 1966 to give earnings-related supplements to the flat-rate unemployment, sickness and widow's allowances; the policy has since been changed and these supplements are to be phased out in 1982.

The next major change in the contribution side came in April 1975 when fully-earnings-related contributions for employees replaced the former combination of flat-rate and graduated contributions. In fact the term 'fully-earnings-related' is misleading since there are both minimum and maximum levels of income on which contributions are based. The early 1970's have been an important period in the development of social security with the Social Security Pensions Act 1975 setting the framework for current pension and disability benefits. However, changes were proposed in the 1980 Budget which need to be taken into account but whose full extent was unknown at the time of going to press.

In November 1970, pensions for those who had been above pension age when the national insurance scheme started were introduced, to be followed in September 1971 by a non-contributory (if relatively low) pension for other people aged over 80.

In April 1971 widows aged between 40 and 50 at the time of their husband's death became eligible for widow's pensions when entitlement to widowed mother's allowance ended. Also in 1971, a radical (although not very costly) Family Income Supplement scheme was introduced. This benefit is different in character from the rest of the scheme, because it is an income *supplement* for full-time earners, as opposed to a form of earnings replacement. It is limited to families with children, where the head is in full time work, and it gives a level of benefit of half the difference between the prescribed levels and the income of the claimant.

Social security and the disabled Benefits for the disabled have figured prominently in the developments of the 1970's. In September 1971 an invalidity pension was introduced for those who had received sickness benefit for six months, plus a small invalidity allowance based on age at the onset of disability. Additionally, a benefit to compensate severely disabled people for the costs of their care, the attendance allowance, was introduced in December 1971. It was later extended at a lower rate to those requiring constant attention *either* by day *or* by night. In addition, people (*except* married women) who cannot go out to work because they spend at least 35 hours a week caring for a severely disabled relative, became eligible from July 1976 to a taxable invalid care allowance.

From January 1976 a taxable mobility allowance was introduced, payable to people unable, or virtually unable, to walk because of physical disablement, extending to all some of the mobility provisions for the disabled which already existed to those eligible for the invalid car.

However, perhaps the most interesting departure from the original conception of the Beveridge scheme was the introduction of non-contributory insurance benefits. The non-contributory invalidity pension was introduced in 1975 and is payable to people of working age who are unable to work and who have been unable to satisfy the contribution condition for invalidity pension. After some delay, and with stringent conditions attached (following years of campaigning by the Disablement Income Group), this was extended to disabled housewives. This benefit was the housewives' non-contributory invalidity pension introduced in November 1977. All these benefits were lower than the SB level or the equivalent contributory benefits and therefore most beneficiaries had *also* to apply for SB. This differential may well change in the lifetime of the Conservative government elected in 1979.

Parallel to this system of benefits are the provisions for war pensioners. Although primarily intended for members of the armed forces, they may also apply to civilians injured by enemy action. In this case the disablement pensions are calculated on the basis of the degree of disablement and there are supplements to the basic levels for unemployability, constant attendance, age, and so on.

It should be noted that those who are disabled at work will be helped under the Industrial Injuries scheme, and that some disablement leads to claims in court, perhaps from an Area Health Authority, which can lead to substantial awards of damages, yet the needs of that particular disabled person will be neither greater nor lesser than the needs of someone disabled by a disease such as multiple sclerosis.

Other forms of financial help   In addition to the basic social security scheme, there is a wide variety of other means-tested benefits, many administered and financed by local authorities, which add significantly to the complexity of the income maintenance provisions (National Consumer Council 1975). Such benefits include free school meals, reduced charges for home helps, grants towards school uniforms and education maintenance allowances. Also relevant are exemptions from NHS charges. This exemption is automatically given to those receiving SB or Family Income Supplement, but others who are poor may also claim. Such charges include dental treatment and prescription charges.

A major anomaly here is the way that a person or family with an income just *above* the line drawn for eligibility for some of these benefits may well, after paying, for example, for school meals, be *worse* off than someone with a slightly lower income who receives free school meals. This phenomenon is sometimes described as 'the poverty trap'!

The continuance of poverty in Britain

Given the range of benefits available for income support, and the expenditure in 1978–9 of £15,441m on social security benefits, how is it that poverty still persists? The major reason, in the terms in which we have defined it, is that the level of National Insurance benefits, at the flat-rate levels, is normally below the corresponding levels of SB. Thus in order *not* to be in poverty a substantial proportion of national insurance beneficiaries must also claim SB to top up inadequate insurance benefits. However, not all those who are eligible for SB do in fact claim it. Those who through ignorance, pride, fear of stigma, or fear of officials do not claim make up the majority of those who continue to live in poverty.

The take-up rate for national insurance benefits is higher than that for means-tested benefits, and it is argued that this reflects the different perceptions of the nature of entitlement (national insurance benefits having been 'paid for' by specific contributions, whereas assistance benefits have not). Hence, it is worrying that the structure of insurance benefits is such as to perpetuate heavy, and in the case of unemployed persons, growing reliance on SB. The structural causes are twofold.

Firstly, the earnings-related supplements to sickness and unemployment benefits have previously ceased after 28 weeks and beneficiaries have then been forced to rely on flat-rate levels of benefit. With the implementation of the Social Security Act 1975, the invalidity benefit, which replaces sickness benefit after 28 weeks, is earnings-related. Current proposals are, however, that the earnings-related supplement will itself be abolished in 1982. Secondly, some of the benefits are themselves of limited duration: for example, unemployment benefit lasts only for one year, after which SB must be claimed (if the claimant is a married woman her husband must make the claim).

In addition, there are certain restrictions on the award of benefit which may mean that a person's actual entitlement may be below his nominal entitlement. In the case of sickness and unemployment benefit, for example, the earnings-related supplement must not, when combined with the flat-rate benefit, raise the level of benefit above 85% of reckonable weekly earnings for the relevant tax year (normally the previous year). For lower earners and in times of inflation this can be important.

Within the SB scheme itself there are restrictions which can be applied to keep benefits down below usual entitlement. A number of so called 'workshy' provisions exist, as does the 'four-week rule' which may limit the receipt of benefit of fit, single men under 45 years of age to four weeks in areas where work is available. Benefit to families where the wage-earners are on strike is likely to be reduced in the early 1980's.

The major limitation to the effectiveness of the SB scheme in bringing people's income up to the poverty line, however, is the level of take-up – that is, the proportion of those eligible for benefit who actually claim it. Average take-up is about 74% and on this basis some £240m of benefit is unclaimed. However, this is by no means the only significant factor. As we have noted, some groups are excluded from entitlement; notable amongst these are those in full-time work.

Only since 1971 with the introduction of Family Income Supplement (FIS) has there been a general income support scheme for those in full-time work. This scheme is however limited to those with dependent children, and the award is limited to *half* the amount by which gross income falls short of the 'prescribed amounts', which are based on the entitlement levels of SB. FIS suffers the disadvantage of all means-tested benefits: low-take up. As with other means-tested benefits, take-up is greater where entitlement is higher, but overall a take-up rate of between 50% and 75% of those eligible for FIS is normally assumed.

New proposals for reform

Two new Social Security Bills were being discussed as this chapter was written. The first (now the Social Security Act 1980) means that pensions will now increase in line with prices (not earnings or prices as before). The long-term rate of SB will be paid after one year (but not to the unemployed). School-leavers' claims to SB can only be made at the end of the holiday following their last term at school. People with capital over £2,000 are excluded from the SB scheme. Full details of all the changes are set out in the *Supplementary Benefits Handbook* (7th edition) published by the DHSS in September 1980.

The second Bill aims to abolish earnings-related supplements by 1982, reduce benefits to strikers and their families, and could lead to lower rates of short-term NI benefits in relation to inflation.

It remains to be seen how these changes will affect the numbers in poverty although the government itself has estimated that these measures will increase the numbers dependent on SB by 100,000.

Conclusions

So far we have attempted to answer the question 'why does poverty – in terms of an income below the appropriate SB entitlement – still exist?' but we should be aware that this phrasing of the question emphasises the effectiveness of the income maintenance system, rather than the underlying *structural causes* of poverty. These causes would include low incomes generally, unemployment and other features which some critics would identify as inherent in a capitalist economy. For these groups, poverty and exploitation are central to the structure of our society, and will be eliminated only by *fundamental structural change* in the nature of society, for example a move to a socialist society.

Our discussion thus far has been mainly in terms of financial indicators of poverty, but poverty, seen as deprivation, is multi-faceted, and one important dimension is health. The link is two-fold: those in poor health are more likely to be poor (see Figure 5.1 which shows the risk of a couple being in poverty when the man is disabled to be much higher than if he is not), and those in poverty are more likely than other groups to suffer poor health. The poor are also likely to be found in poorer-quality housing, again with implications for health. This aspect of poverty must be of real concern to the day-to-day work of those in the helping professions, but especially to nurses.

SUMMARY OF MAJOR SOCIAL SECURITY AND TAX BENEFITS

National Insurance   The main categories of National Insurance Benefits are retirement pensions, sickness benefit, invalidity benefit (which follows sickness benefit) and unemployment benefit.

Retirement Pensions are payable at the normal retirement ages of 65 for men and 60 for women, at the single person's or the married couple's rate, with additions for dependants. The provision of retirement pensions can either be wholly through the state scheme, or through a combination of state and private pension schemes.

Sickness Benefit   Sickness benefit is paid for up to 28 weeks during a spell of incapacity for work. It is then replaced by invalidity benefit. Sickness benefit is not paid for the first three days of incapacity. An earnings-related supplement may be payable from the thirteenth day of a period of interruption of employment to people under minimum pension age, who have paid Class I Contributions, for up to six months in any one period of interruption of employment, but this will be discontinued in 1982. (A proposal is currently under discussion whereby most employers would be made responsible for paying employees for the first eight weeks of sickness, making this benefit liable to tax.

Invalidity Benefit Invalidity benefit is paid to a person who has received sickness benefit for 28 weeks and is still unable to go to work as a result of sickness or injury.

Unemployment Benefit Unemployment benefit is payable for up to one year in any period of interruption of employment. It is not paid for the first three days, or for single isolated days. An earnings-related supplement is payable on the same basis as that for sickness benefit, but this also will be discontinued in 1982.

Maternity Benefit A lump-sum maternity grant is payable to most mothers on the basis of *their own* or *their husband's national insurance contributions*. From 1982, this will be paid to *all* irrespective of contribution record.

A *maternity allowance* is paid to women who have been paying full national insurance contributions (although it can be paid at a lower rate if the contribution conditions are not met). It is normally payable from 11 weeks before the expected week of confinement, until the sixth week following the expected week, or the actual confinement of this is later. In October 1980, the government issued a consultative document setting out plans for the future of maternity benefits but no decisions had been taken as this book went to press.

Death Grant A lump-sum death grant is payable on the death of a male contributor, his wife, child or widow, or on the death of a female contributor, her husband, child or widower. The rate of grant depends on the age of the deceased – with a lower rate for children in comparison to adults.

Industrial injuries Running in parallel with the NI scheme is the Industrial Injuries scheme which provides injury and disablement benefits. This scheme is not described in detail as it is currently under review.

Benefits for widows and their children

Widow's Allowance The widow's allowance is payable for the first 26 weeks after the husband's death. It is at a higher rate than other NI benefits, and carries both an earnings-related supplement and additions for children.

Widowed Mother's Allowance This is payable when widow's allowance ends if, and so long as, the widow has in her family a qualifying child under the child benefit age limits.

Widow's pension Widow's pensions are payable to widows who are 40 years old or over when their husbands die or when their entitlement to widowed mother's allowance ceases. Payment of a pension starts as soon as they stop receiving widow's allowance or widowed mother's allowance. Payment continues at the same rate irrespective of earnings until the widow remarries or dies or begins to draw retirement pension.

Child's Special Allowance A child's special allowance is payable to a mother on the death of her former husband if the marriage has been dissolved or annulled and the former husband had continued to contribute to the support of the children.

National insurance non-contributory benefits

Despite the fact that considerable emphasis is placed on the contributory basis of the National Insurance Scheme, two non-contributory but 'insurance' benefits (in that they are not taxable and not means-tested) have emerged in the 1970's. These parallel the contributory benefits but are at a lower rate than their contributory equivalent, ie. approximately 60%.

Non-contributory Invalidity Pension – NCIP This is payable to people of working age who are unable to work and who have not satisfied the contribution conditions for national insurance invalidity pension (for example, by never having been in the workforce).

This benefit is non-taxable but is subject to an earnings limit, and a husband's entitlement may be affected by his wife's earnings, and serves primarily to reduce its recipients' reliance on SB, although it also carries with it credited national insurance contributions. From November 1977 disabled housewives became eligible for the

Housewives' NCIP This carries two conditions:
  1 that they are incapable of working, and
  2 that they are incapable of performing their normal household duties.

Other non-contributory benefits

Attendance Allowance A weekly allowance payable to people who are severely disabled, physically and mentally, and who for six months or more have required from another person, frequent attention or continual supervision by day and at night. A lower rate is payable to people requiring such attention by day *or* at night. The benefit is tax free and not means-tested.

Mobility Allowance A taxable cash benefit for severely disabled adults under pensionable age and severely disabled children aged 5 years or more.

The criterion of eligibility is that the person is 'unable or virtually unable' to walk because of physical disablement and is likely to remain so for at least a year. It is payable in addition to other social security benefits.

Invalid Care Allowance Became payable in July 1976 to people who cannot go out to work because they spend at least 35 hours a week caring for a severely disabled relative who receives an attendance allowance, *or* a constant attendance allowance under the industrial injuries or war pensions schemes. It is not payable in addition to some other social security benefits and, in general, married women cannot qualify for the invalid care allowance. It is taxable and subject to an earnings limit.

Child Benefit Child benefit is a non-contributory, tax-free benefit for each child, to the parent (normally the mother) or anyone else responsible for a child under 16 (or under 19 if still at school full-time).

Guardian's Allowance A non-contributory benefit available to a person who takes an orphan child into the family.

Child Benefit Increase Lone parents, or anyone bringing up children alone may qualify for an additional amount in addition to the child benefit for the first or only child. In normal circumstances, the amount is reviewed annually.

Further details of all social security benefits can be found in DHSS leaflet FB2 *Which Benefit?* which is available from local DHSS offices, and in the current edition of the Supplementary Benefits Handbook.

Reliefs in the tax system

Tax Allowances   Single parents qualify for an additional personal allowance which, with their single person's allowance, equals the married man's tax allowance.

Dependent Relative's Allowance   A dependent relative's allowance is due to a taxpayer who maintains, wholly or partially, either (a) an aged or infirm relative, or (b) his or his wife's separated, divorced or widowed mother. The relative's income must be below the limit of the basic National Insurance Retirement Pension for the full allowance to be given, and is reduced, pound for pound, by the relative's excess over the income limit.

Daughter's Services Allowance   The daughter's services allowance may be claimed by an aged or infirm taxpayer who maintains a son or daughter upon whose services he or his wife are dependent.

Housekeeper Allowance   This may be claimed by a widow or widower who has a resident housekeeper.

Blind Person's Allowance   This is paid to a registered blind taxpayer but is reduced by the amount of any tax-free blindness disability pension.

Further details of these and other reliefs are available from any Inland Revenue Tax Office.

References

Abel-Smith B. & Townsend P. (1965) *The Poor and the Poorest.*
   Occasional Papers on Social Administration 17. London: Bell
Beveridge W. (1942) *Social Insurance and Allied Services.* Cmd
   6404. London: HMSO

Booth W. (1970) *In Darkness England and the Way Out*. London: Knight

DHSS/Supplementary Benefits Commission (1978) *Take-up of Supplementary Benefits*. London: HMSO

Finer M. (1974) *Report of the Committee on One-Parent families*. Cmnd 5629. London: HMSO

Layard R., Piachaud D. & Steward M. (1978) *The Causes of Poverty. Background Paper No. 5, Royal Commission on the Distribution of Income and Wealth*. London: HMSO

National Consumer Council (1975) *Means-tested Benefits*. London: National Consumer Council

Rowntree B. S. (1901) *Poverty: A Study of Town Life*. London: Macmillan

Chapter 6

The National Health Service

Judith Allsop

The relationship between health and welfare services

The health and personal social services in Britain provide a range of caring and curing services – and to a lesser extent a preventive service – for individuals and families. The services are operated by professional and administrative staffs with a wide range of skills. Of these, the nurse is a member of the largest professional group. The services have a common purpose, in that they are concerned to help people with problems of ill health and handicap, which may or may not be combined with difficult social and environmental situations.

This chapter aims to describe the role and structure of the National Health Service (NHS). The following chapter examines the Social Service Departments and the role of voluntary agencies, which may provide alternative or complementary sources of care. In discussing these provisions, it is important to remember there is often a gap between what the services are *meant* to achieve and their *actual* achievements, which may be considerably less. The gap may be due to shortage of resources, or to the quality of those operating or organising such services, or it may be that the problems facing clients or patients are beyond the scope of the service. Social or medical problems associated with unemployment or inadequate housing may be the result of the broader economic and political policies discussed in earlier chapters.

The administrative structures which have developed to provide health and personal social services have differing histories which have influenced their present form of organisation.

Health services are provided through organisations with direct responsibility to the Secretary of State for Health and Social Services, while personal social services are provided through local authority (and elected) Social Service Committees, responsible to the elected local authority itself. This has created what W. J. M. Mackenzie (1979) has called 'a deep underlying fissure in English institutions'. Decision making is different in the two services, and this in turn affects those who work in the services as well as those who receive them. Collaboration between the services is made difficult, although they pursue the broadly common aims of meeting social need. Attempts to bring the health and social services closer together is a recurrent theme in both this chapter and the next, as the division is often artificial, yet can create problems for the community nurse as well as for the nurse concerned with discharging patients from hospital.

The Report of a working party set up by the DHSS and the Personal Social Services Council (*Collaboration in Community Care* 1978) found there was often a lack of contact between health and social services, and gaps in the knowledge of each other's functions. In addition, their work is organised very differently. Social services departments work in area teams with many different types of client. The health service is divided into primary care which provides first-level general health care in local geographical areas and secondary or specialist care which is clinically based and often caters for patients from wider areas. As Harbridge (1980) points out, health service staff usually work relatively fast, making decisions for their patients (often including value judgements) and provide treatment that is very often obvious in its effect. Social workers, on the other hand, may allow their clients to determine the pace at which they work, stress non-judgemental attitudes and may have less obvious methods of help at their disposal. Although the different organisation and geographical context of health and of social services provision is important, it is equally important to realise that differences in outlook and training between social workers and nurses are also crucial.

At the level of the professional worker relationship, if a social worker and a health visitor are both visiting a client, then each should be aware of the aims and goals of the other. The social worker, for instance, may not understand the degree of mobility that can reasonably be expected from a disabled person. Similarly, a community-based social worker may have a deeper knowledge of problems affecting the area (vandalism, for example) that could be relevant to the individual's health. It is important that each worker's role should be well defined, and understood by the workers in all areas. A lack of such understanding can have particularly dangerous results in cases of suspected non-accidental injury or the neglected elderly person.

The district nurse visits patients with an 'illness' problem (eg. a leg ulcer), and the social worker those with a 'social' problem (eg. a mentally handicapped child in the family), but the unique contribution of the health visitor may be her contact with a wide range of normal families, giving her a solid base from which to help families with a range of problems spreading across the traditional health and welfare boundaries. Indeed, during the social worker strikes of 1979, it was the health visitor in many areas who found herself dealing with complex problems which she would otherwise have handed over to the social worker.

It is worth noting that the organisation of health and social services is slightly different in Wales and Scotland from that in England, although the issues relating to service provision are, of course, similar. There are, however, fundamental differences in the structure of services in Northern Ireland, where health and social services are operated together under a joint Health and Social Services Board.

In the remainder of this chapter the focus is on the National Health Service, and on the issues which have dominated policy debates, affecting both the role and structure of the service. A more detailed chronological account of this development is available in *The NHS, the First Phase* (Watkin 1978).

Dilemmas in the NHS: an overview

The NHS, as it was established in 1948, embodied three new principles: firstly, medical care was to be provided free at the point of service, to those who presented themselves as being in need; secondly, this right to individual care was to be available to the whole population; and thirdly, central government became directly responsible for policy and management of the supply of health care – curative, caring and preventive. To many people this constituted a radical change from the past and placed the health service at the centre of post-war reconstruction. Prior to 1948, medical care had been free at the point of service only to those working men insured under the Insurance Act 1911 or with the many private insurance schemes available. The pattern of care was uneven and fragmented, and this had been forcibly driven home to central government when it took over medical services as part of the war effort in 1940.

These three principles have shaped the provision of health services since 1948 and have not been seriously challenged, although they have been somewhat eroded by rising prescription and dental charges, and increasingly so in the late 1970's and early 1980's. There have been differences of emphasis between the political parties in relation to priorities in health care as well as in relation to the limits of State responsibility. The role of the private sector and the question of how best to administer this expensive and unwieldly health service are debated within and between the political parties. However, the basic individual right to health care for the whole population has yet to be challenged.

Ever since the inception of the NHS there has been a debate about the rising costs of medical care. In 1949, NHS expenditure was 4·0% of the Gross Domestic Product, and by 1977 this had risen to 5·6%. In money terms, the cost of the NHS has risen from £433m to £6897m in the same period (Chester 1979). The rise in expenditure has been particularly rapid since the 1960's, as can be seen from Figure 6.1 which shows rising expenditure in all aspects of health and welfare services, but particularly in Area Health Authority expenditure of which acute hospital services are the major element. These rising expenditures reflect growing aspirations and expectations by patients and health care professions; they also reflect technological developments which are inevitably expensive as they become more and more commonly used (eg. renal dialysis, intensive care units).

Many would argue that the health service is under-funded, and, indeed, in relation to many other comparable industrialised societies the United Kingdom spends a smaller proportion of its national wealth on health care (OHE 1979). This means that quite legitimate demands may go unmet or are subject to long delays.

The role of the NHS

The rising costs of health care led, in the 1970's, to a fundamental questioning of the role of the NHS. In 1947 the stated aim was to 'secure improvements in the mental and physical health of the nation

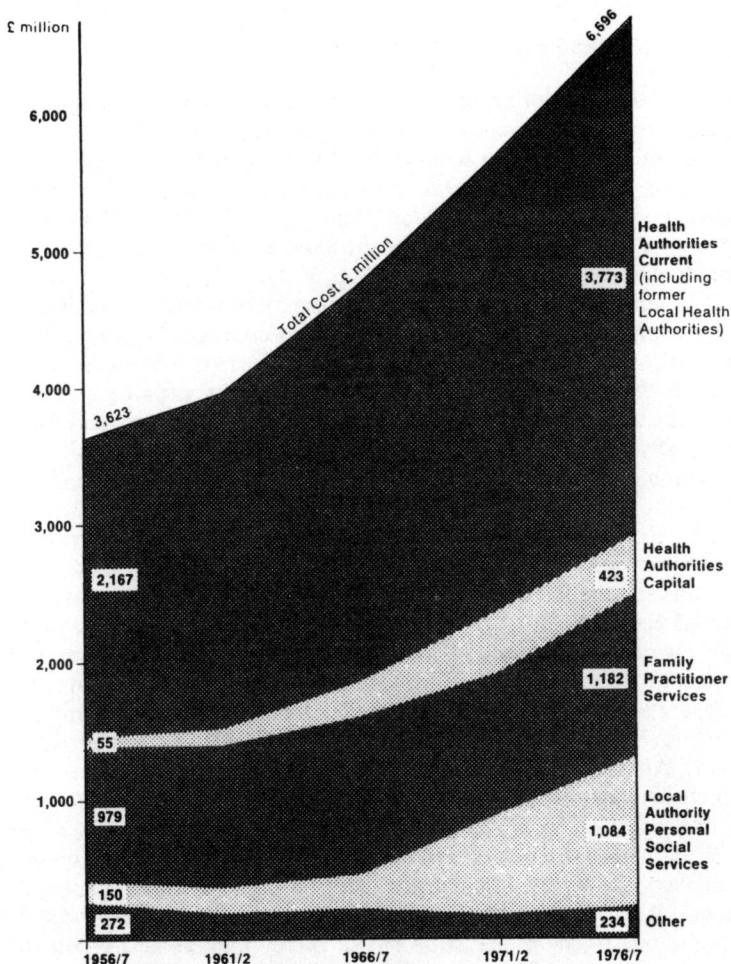

£ million

6,696

6,000

5,000

Health Authorities Current (including former Local Health Authorities) — 3,773

4,000

3,623

3,000

2,167

Health Authorities Capital — 423

2,000

Family Practitioner Services — 1,182

55

1,000

979

Local Authority Personal Social Services — 1,084

150

272

Other — 234

1956/7   1961/2   1966/7   1971/2   1976/7

Total Cost £ million

Notes

1 Expenditure is shown at November 1976 prices.

2 Over the years there have been variations in the nature and coverage of the services. The chart therefore shows the broad trend only.

3 Separate accounts were not kept for England and Wales before 1967/8. This chart is on an England and Wales basis over the whole period in order to present a consistent picture.

Fig 6.1 Growth of expenditure on health and personal social services 1956/57 to 1976/77: England and Wales (from *DHSS Annual Report 1977*. Reproduced by permission of the Controller of Her Majesty's Stationery Office)

through the prevention, diagnosis and treatment of illness and for that purpose to provide or secure the effective provision of services'. Health, in this view, was seen as the absence of illness and the NHS was part of a wider programme to eradicate Disease along with Ignorance, Squalor, Idleness and Want (Beveridge 1942). Beveridge envisaged that spending on the health services would decrease as the health of the nation improved.

The aims of the NHS as set out in the 1979 Royal Commission Report provide interesting similarities and contrasts: it states 'The NHS should encourage and assist individuals to remain healthy, provide equality of entitlement to health services, provide a broad range of services to a high standard, provide equality of access to these services, provide a service free at the time of use, satisfy the reasonable expectations of users, remain a national service responsive to local needs'.

The Commission's view is that the aim should be to provide a health service free at the point of consumption, but they also emphasised the importance of preventing disease. This is seen as a shared responsibility – 'everybody's business' (DHSS: *Prevention and Health* 1977), and if it is to be taken seriously implies an increase in the proportion of the budget spent on preventive health measures. In 1975 only 0·42% of the NHS budget was spent on preventive health (DHSS: *Priorities in Health and Welfare Services* 1977). Also implicit here is the need to change attitudes to life styles which promote ill health (eg. tobacco smoking, excessive alcohol drinking etc).

What is also interesting about the Royal Commission's views on the role of the NHS is the stress given to equality of entitlement and access. It hardly occurred to the legislators in 1946 that this would ever be one of the major concerns of policy makers and prove so difficult to realise. There are still large differences in the health of people in different social classes. To take just one indicator, the Court Report (1976) points out that children in Social Class V are twice as likely to die between the end of the first month and the end of the first year of life as a child born to parents in Social Classes I and II: 'Twice as many children of unskilled workers die in the first month of life as children of professional workers and the gap between the social classes in this respect has been widening steadily for 25 years. Two and a half times more children die in Classes IV and V than in Classes I and II, of certain infectious diseases. Children still die in our lifetime for nineteenth century reasons'. A large part of these differences is caused by social and environmental factors, but lack of equality of access plays a part. There are many ways in which people in Social Classes IV and V make less use of the NHS even though they have higher mortality rates. This is particularly marked when the uptake of preventive services is examined (eg. cervical smears or preventive dentistry). The wider factors contributing to these variations in mortality are even more difficult to influence as they reflect intrinsic inequalities within society which medical care alone cannot reverse.

In its two final aims the Royal Commission implied that the NHS cannot satisfy all expectations: demands are infinite and resources increasingly limited. Choices must be made, and this is also 'everybody's business' – at all levels of service provision – which is discussed in Chapter 9.

Illsley (1976) has suggested that the emphasis of the NHS since 1946 has moved

from:	*to:*
illness	health
treatment	prevention
cure	care
disease	behaviour producing disease
individual treatment	population as a unit of treatment
illness as a concern of the medical profession	health as the business of everyone
right to treatment	duty to remain healthy

The nurse, whether working in the community or in hospital, may well feel that these changes in emphasis, as suggested by Illsey, are slow to take effect and that treatment and cure, for example, have resources and a status which the preventive and caring work of the NHS still lacks. There is now a greater divergency of opinion about the proper role of the NHS and how better health can be achieved than perhaps at any time since the mid-19th century.

Rising costs have led to questions on priorities within the NHS being asked by those who allocate the resources which the Service uses. Answers have been sought by attempting to change the administrative structure to achieve greater efficiency (value for money) and effectiveness (more appropriate care). Large numbers of commissions and committees have looked at the structure of the NHS and at the functioning of particular aspects of it. Further structural change is planned for the 1980's, but problems remain intractable – there can be no 'perfect' structure, for the task of the NHS is complex and its organisation large, employing nearly one million people.

Many organisational dilemmas facing the NHS have been 'solved' in different ways at different times; however, a 'solution' often creates new sets of problems. The basic structure was laid down in 1948 and we now move to examine it in some detail.

The tripartite structure of the NHS: 1948–1974

The tripartite structure established in 1948 was so called because the services were divided into three separate parts, organised and financed in different ways. Firstly, hospitals other than teaching hospitals were run by Hospital Management Committees consisting of members appointed by the Minister of Health, some of whom were lay people and others were from the hospital medical staff. The committees were responsible to one of the 13 Regional Hospital Boards which, in turn, were responsible to the Minister. Resources were allocated to the Regional Hospital Boards on an historic basis (ie. based on allocations made in previous years rather than in accordance with any rational measurement of need), and the Regional Boards allocated moneys to each Hospital Management Committee. Teaching hospitals were organised differently, having Boards of Governors and being financed directly by the Ministry: they tended to obtain a major part of the resources.

Secondly, local authorities (counties and county boroughs) had health departments which provided a variety of health services under the direction of the Medical Officer of Health: these included district nursing, midwifery services, health visiting, home helps, ambulances, and other preventive health services. Some local authorities ran their health and welfare services as a combined department. The quality and quantity of the services provided by different local authorities varied considerably, as, indeed, happens now with social services and other locally-administered services.

The third arm of the health services consisted of the services provided by general practitioners, opticians and pharmacists under contract to the NHS. These contracts were managed by Executive Councils which included both representatives of the professions and lay appointees, and covered roughly the same geographical areas as counties and county boroughs.

The three parts of the health services provided different *types* of care:

(a) specialist care in the hospitals;
(b) community services in people's own homes; and
(c) a community-based first-line diagnostic, treatment and referral service operated by GPs, increasingly aided by attached community health staff.

This division of services was based on history and compromise rather than logic. Divisions grew up between doctors working in hospital medicine, general practice and local health authorities (and indeed between hospital nursing and community nursing), during the 19th century. This, in part, was due to the increasing importance of hospitals as centres of clinical practice, research and education.

These divisions in the provision of health care were the concern of the Dawson Committee as early as 1920. This committee called for an administratively-integrated health service, with preventive and curative services brought together in a network of primary and secondary health centres. The secondary centres would be based on existing general hospitals which would be linked with teaching hospitals. Administration would be carried out by largely elected authorities, under a Medical Officer.

The Dawson report, and other similar recommendations foundered on opposition from the medical profession. There was hostility to any form of local control of hospitals, and family doctors were opposed to working for a salary. The tripartite system agreed in 1946 was therefore a compromise reached in order to accommodate medical interests, and as a result two issues in health care were side-stepped: one was the question of continuity of care, and the second was the issue of central control versus the responsiveness of health authorities to local needs.

Under the tripartite structure the Ministry of Health was to be a 'laissez-faire' department; executive powers were to be devolved to the Regional Hospital Boards and to the Hospital Management Committees. Little attempt was made to enforce national policies, and Hospital Management Committees were not responsive to local pressures. Crossman (1972) called them 'self-perpetuating oligarchies'.

These two issues were to recur in the various reports leading to reorganisation of the NHS in 1974, although the solutions proposed differed. The build-up began with the Report of the Porritt Committee (1962), which was set up by doctors. Next, and perhaps more important, was the Labour Government's first Green Paper published in 1968 when Kenneth Robinson was Minister of Health (a Green Paper is a discussion paper published by the government to encourage comments from interested parties, as opposed to a White Paper which usually outlines action the government proposes to take). The 1968 Green Paper received a hostile reception and was followed by a second Green Paper in 1970, by which time Richard Crossman was Secretary of State at the newly created Department of Health and Social Security. With the change of government, the Conservatives published a Consultative Document in 1971, when Keith Joseph was Secretary of State, and the 1974 reorganisation was based on this 1971 document. Before discussing these changes, the altering context of health care provision between 1948 and 1974 needs to be examined.

The changing context of health care

Firstly, the pattern of mortality and morbidity has changed over the last century particularly in the latter half. The main causes of death are no longer infectious diseases: heart disease, cancer and stroke have replaced them. Morbidity, which is the prevalence of illness, is more difficult to measure, but in terms of hospital admissions, respiratory and digestive diseases alone accounted for 25% of admissions in 1972. In terms of time spent in hospital, diseases of the heart and circulation took first place during the 1970's. Mental illness is also a major problem: 44% of hospital beds are occupied by the mentally ill. In general practice, 400-450 consultations out of every 2,500 relate to chronic disease and disability. Dental caries is the most prevalent disease of all (DHSS: Prevention and Health 1976).

As McKeown (1976) argues, the causal factors in these illnesses and deaths are related to complex combinations of behavioural, environmental and genetic factors, and the application of the simple disease model of illness does not help us to understand or prevent them.

Secondly, as was noted in earlier chapters, there have been important changes in the age and sex structure of the population, with far-reaching consequences in relation to health and social problems. For example, there are larger numbers of very elderly people, especially elderly women, in both absolute and relative terms than there were in 1948 and, as all nurses will know, this is a group which makes particularly high demands on the health services.

These factors have led many people to question the appropriateness of the health service structure and its ordering of priorities. Should hospital medicine, for example, continue to take the major proportion of NHS spending when the need for services which care rather than cure is so great? Should the NHS be a 'sickness service' or should more be spent on preventive health measures? (Owen 1978). The pressures to increase resources for acute medicine are intense. New technologies such as renal dialysis, transplant surgery, body scanners and new drug therapies have helped to raise public and professional expectations, and to focus attention on the hospital, and there have been further pressures to distribute specialist services more evenly throughout the country.

Weaknesses of the tripartite structure   Criticisms of the tripartite structure can be summarised as follows:

(a) lack of continuity of care;
(b) lack of an adequate basis for planning nationally determined priorities;
(c) lack of an adequate management structure to achieve effective and efficient allocation of resources;
(d) lack of accountability to the consumer; and
(e) dominance of the acute hospital, leading to a lack of emphasis on the caring and preventive aspects of medicine.

Two major factors lie behind the perception of these issues as 'problems': one is the development of the policy of community care, and the second is the idea that better management and planning within *larger* institutions and over *larger* areas of administration will lead to greater value for money in health services provision.

Community care and the need for efficiency

The move towards a policy for the development of community care stemmed from the Royal Commission on the Mental Health Services (1959). Hospital and local health authorities were urged to adopt policies which would maintain people in their own homes or in their local community, through the provision of day hospitals, out-patient facilities in local hospitals, hostels, day centres and support at home from general practitioners, as well as from social work and nursing staff. This was felt to be a 'better' way of providing care as well as being cheaper: costs of in-patient care are high. During the 1960's books such as Peter Townsend's *The Last Refuge* (1964), Barbara Robb's *Sans Everything* (1967) and Pauline Morris' *Put Away* (1969) underlined the poor quality of much of the care offered in large custodial institutions for groups such as the elderly and the mentally handicapped. The later enquiries into the Ely (1969), Whittingham (1972) and Farleigh (1971) Hospitals, with their accounts of cruelty, neglect, inadequate staffing and facilities, helped to encourage the philosophy of community care as an alternative to care in the large hospital.

One of the difficulties in achieving a radical change in this direction lay in the problem of defining clearly the meaning of the term 'community care'. The term has been used in at least three different ways, and is still open to discussion. Firstly, it can mean care by health or social service workers in residential accommodation on a smaller scale than the large institution, and within people's own local community. Examples would include small residential homes for the mentally handicapped, or sheltered accommodation for the elderly. Secondly, community care can also mean services provided in people's existing homes, by nursing or social work staff – such as district nursing or meals on wheels. Thirdly, community care can mean care by the community through the support systems which are usually taken for granted, but which in fact provide the vast majority of care for those in need. This support system includes primarily the family, but also neighbourly help and voluntary help. Surprisingly little is known about this 'hidden labour force' (Taylor 1979) and the factors which encourage neighbourliness and mutual support systems in caring (Abrams 1980). Still less is known about the interaction between the three types of community care outlined above. Nevertheless, the policy remains a central feature of government strategy as well as having played an important part of the discussions leading up to the 1974 NHS reorganisation. This was one reason why the need for continuity of care between hospital and community health services, and between health and social services, was stressed in the 1974 reorganisation.

Also stressed was the need for greater efficiency in the allocation and use of resources in health. In the 1960's, ways of monitoring services, and policies aiming to provide a wide range of hospital services in larger institutions or over wider catchment areas were developed. The Hospital Plan (MoH 1962) established a 'bed norm', ie. a recommended number of beds per 1,000 population which should be provided for a range of specialities. This 'norm' was to be used to allocate resources. A similar plan was prepared by local authorities for community health and welfare services (MoH 1963).

Another measure aimed at greater efficiency, and linked to the Hospital Plan, with its plans for a renewal of hospital building, was the idea of the District General Hospital. It was argued that large hospitals, serving a population of about 250,000 and providing a comprehensive range of specialisms, would bring economies of scale and provide centres of excellence for the areas they served. These advantages were seen to be more important than accessibility for patients. However, when public expenditure cuts forced a reduction in the amount of hospital rebuilding that was to be allowed, these arguments were forgotten, and the concept of the smaller and adaptable 'nucleus hospital' was introduced.

Arguments for a larger administrative area were to play an important part in the discussions over the reorganisation of local government as well as the health services in the 1970's.

The NHS 1974–1980

It was suggested earlier in this chapter that there is always a tension between government's wish to control services from the centre in order to implement national policies, national standards of care, and national norms for equality of provision, and the need to have services which are responsive to local pressures. There are more elderly people in Bournemouth than in Milton Keynes, for example, and the pattern of services in the two areas should reflect this difference. The 1974 NHS reorganisation attempted to solve this dilemma by creating larger units of administration. Area Health Authorities (AHAs) were established, which administered hospital *and* community health services in areas *coterminous* (ie. having the same geographical boundaries) with the newly-reorganised local government structure. In addition, Community Health Councils were set up, which enabled the local consumers to react to management of their health services.

The National Health Service Reorganisation Act 1973 established the new structure. Responsible to the DHSS were to be 14 Regional Health Authorities (RHAs) and 90 AHAs. Most AHAs were further sub-divided into Districts for management purposes, although there were to be some single district areas; There were 205 Districts, each with an average population of 230,000. The RHAs were responsible for: strategic planning, major building, some specialised clinical services and monitoring the services and planning proposals of AHAs. The AHAs had a dual responsibility; assessing the needs of the area for community health and hospital services *and* providing services to meet those needs. The District was the operational administrative unit, responsible for the actual day-to-day running of the services.

The freedom of action of the AHA was constrained by the amount of the financial allocation received from the RHA. A further constraint, from 1976, was government insistence that NHS spending be kept within strict financial cost limits. Other centrally-determined policies (eg. on staffing) provide further constraints.

A detailed description of the 1974 structure can be found in Ruth Levitt's book *The Reorganisation of the NHS* (1976) but a simple chart of the structure is shown in Figure 6.2. The major principles involved in the new structure were as follows:

(a) a new planning system was established which involved the setting of priorities and expenditure limits *centrally* and their implementation *locally*.

(b) the co-ordination of community and hospital services with

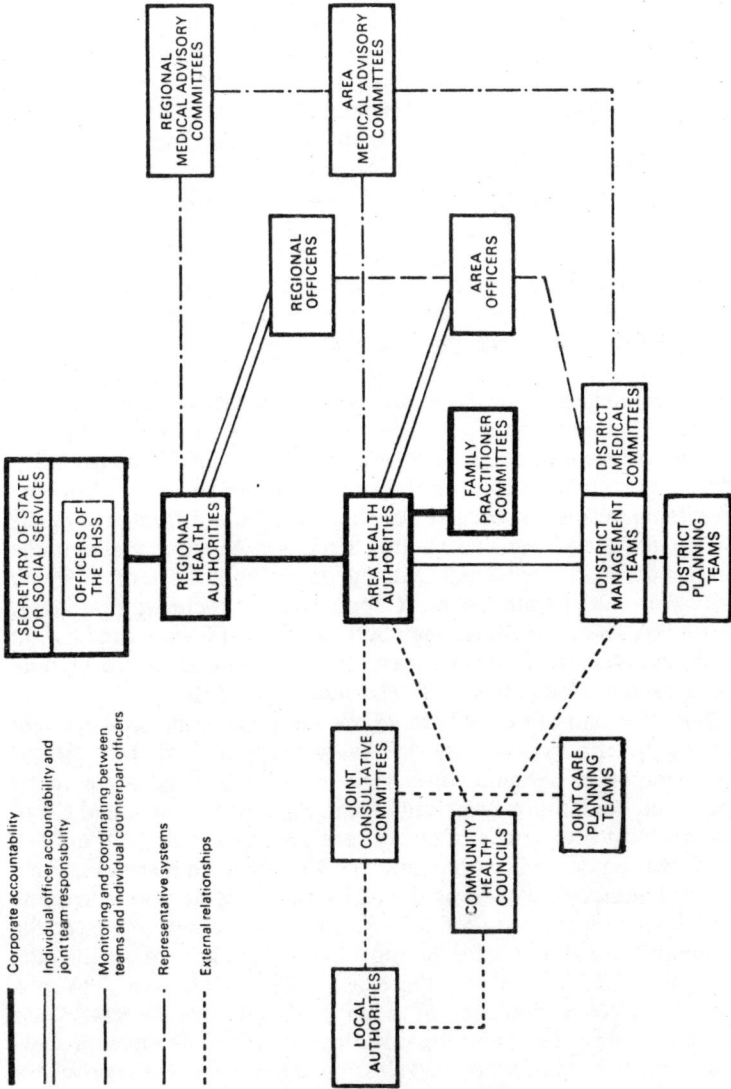

Fig 6.2 Framework of the NHS structure in England (from *The NHS Reorganisation* 1979. Reproduced by kind permission of the Office of Health Economics)

local authority social services and educational provision was stressed. Joint Consultative Committees were set up to ensure that NHS and local government professional and lay managers met regularly.

(c) The operational management of the services was made the responsibility of multidisciplinary management teams, including the District Management Team. A few of the members of the Health Authorities were drawn from the major health professions – doctors and nurses. Furthermore, a series of professional advisory committees (eg. medical, nursing) were created to advise the Health Authorities. Members of the main professions were thus involved in decision making at all levels.

On the management side, the aim was for consensus management. Agreement had to be reached in collective decisions at each level before the decisions could be passed upwards in the decision-making chain. This principle was of great importance to the nursing profession because it became for the first time a formal part of the management and decision-making structure. Most crucial was the nurse member of the District Management Team, the level at which there were no lay management appointees as there were at RHA and AHA level. The other members of the DMT were the District Administrator, the District Treasurer and three doctors, (a hospital consultant, a GP and the District Community Physician).

A further aim of the 1974 reorganisation was to increase accountability to the consumers. AHAs were appointed, but elected members of local authorities were included among those to be appointed, and, much more important, the newly-constituted Community Health Councils (CHCs) were set up in each District. The CHC was made up of approximately 30 appointed members, some by local authorities, a few by the AHA and yet others were to come from local voluntary organisations. The CHC was to represent the community and especially the most vulnerable groups such as the mentally handicapped and the elderly. The CHCs were given a budget to cover the cost of a full-time salaried Secretary and premises. They were to be consulted as part of the planning process and, in particular, over hospital closures. They were also to provide a source of advice and information for the general public, as well as acting as a pressure group in relation to health services in the District. In other words, they would be reacting to management on behalf of the managed.

In 1976, only two years after reorganisation, a Royal Commission was set up 'to consider in the interests of both patients and of those who work in the NHS the best use and management of finance and manpower resource of the NHS'. The Commission was appointed, with Sir Alec Merrison as Chairman, by the Labour Government of 1974–1979, at a time when the NHS was under attack, and at a time when, following the uncertainties of reorganisation, morale within the NHS was low.

The Commission reported in 1979 and this was followed in December of that year by the government's consultative document *Patients First*. The dissatisfaction with the NHS that had led to the appointment of the Royal Commission arose from concern with a number of issues which were troubling those working within the NHS as well as the public at large. Before considering the consultative document these issues will now be discussed: they included:

(a) resource allocation to less affluent regions;
(b) resource allocation to vulnerable patient groups, such as the elderly, the mentally ill, and the mentally handicapped;
(c) collaboration between the health and social services; and
(d) industrial relations.

Resource allocation

The distribution of health resources between regions is unequal in a number of ways. For example, there are great variations in the numbers of general practitioners and dentists per head of population. In addition, the number and range of hospitals, the location of teaching hospitals and the range of medical specialisms available vary widely. The number of hospital beds and the range and extent of community nursing services also vary greatly. The reasons for this inequality are largely historical. The claim for resources made by Regions has been based on past allocation, and teaching hospitals have traditionally made major claims based on their requirements for teaching and research. Inequality occurs not only in relation to different levels of provision: morbidity and mortality rates also vary.

This tends to show an inverse relationship to the resources available (Hart 1971). Those Regions in the country which are *worst* off in terms of the supply of medical care are just those Regions which produce above average *demand*. These demands are linked to health needs, coming from the most deprived parts of the country, with mortality and morbidity closely linked to social class.

The Resources Allocation Working Party (RAWP) was set up in 1975 and first reported in 1976. Its task was to recommend a basis for future regional and area distribution, to ensure that resources were equitably and efficiently distributed according to relative need. The recommendations for capital and current spending over the following ten years were based on a formula which attempted to take into account objective measures of relative need.

The RAWP approach has been widely criticised, both on technical grounds (Carrier 1978) and also because of its implications for those regions (especially those with a high proportion of teaching hospitals) which stand to lose through reallocation. In London, the demand for resources made by the teaching hospitals can have a draining effect on the resources available for community health services and smaller hospitals in that District.

Technical criticisms include that the formula uses mortality rates rather than morbidity as a measure of need, and does not make allowances for other complementary services, such as the quality of the general practitioner service or the extent of local authority social services provision. However, it is technically difficult to produce a formula which all would accept. The formula adopted only concerns allocations from the DHSS to Regions; each RHA is encouraged to adopt the national formula for the purpose of making allocations to its own AHAs, so RAWP does not allow for the striking inequalities *within* regions. The RHA makes decisions on allocations to Areas. A second criticism has been that RAWP takes insufficient account of the expenses of 'centres of excellence', so that where these are found in large numbers, as in London, other services may be particularly short of resources.

The idea of reallocating resources to those regions which were previously seriously underfinanced is a good one; the problem has been that the RAWP proposals have been implemented during a period of very slow growth in public expenditure and a period of rapid inflation. Firstly, under the Labour administration and then under the Conservative government, regions such as the four Thames Regions and the Oxford Region that have been favoured in the past have had to reduce expenditure sharply and quickly in order to divert funds to regions such as those in the north of England. Such a reduction, in a period of rising salary bills, has inevitably led to the closure of beds and even hospitals, as well as to reductions in the training of hospital and community nurses. These measures have not been planned but have often been rushed through with consequent bad effects upon the morale and creativity of NHS staff, as readers may well know from personal experience, and this in turn has had a detrimental effect upon patient care. This exercise in 'positive discrimination' has forced the NHS to debate the hard choices that have to be made between quality and equality, but has shown more clearly than before the extent of the gross under-funding in many Regions.

Allocation to groups needing care   A second issue in the debate about positive discrimination has been concerned with the development of services for particular groups who need caring as well as curing, and who have tended to be the 'cinderellas' of the NHS: the elderly, the mentally ill, the mentally handicapped and the disabled. The elderly occupy 49% of psychiatric beds, and over half the non-psychiatric beds in hospitals; recent demographic trends suggest that demands from these groups will grow. Within the NHS these groups have less status than the acutely ill, as demonstrated, for example, by the strong competition for consultant posts in surgery compared with the shortage of applicants for consultant posts in geriatrics. One could also point to the ratio of qualified to unqualified nursing staff in mental handicap nursing compared with medical wards in acute general hospitals.

The DHSS consultative documents *Priorities in the Health and Welfare Services* (1976) and *The Way Forward* (1977) represent attempts by the Department to take the lead in moving from an emphasis on curative services to an emphasis on the caring services, but because of the reduction in growth of public expenditure the changes have been difficult to bring about. It has, in fact, proved easier to move towards reducing geographical inequalities than towards reducing inequalities between client groups. One reason for this is that decisions on regional resource allocations are taken centrally but decisions on reallocating between patient groups are decided locally, giving a higher possibility of professional in-fighting! It has been easier, therefore, to establish differing percentage increases in expenditure, than it has been to plan to increase the expenditure on a particular client group (Carrier 1978).

Nevertheless, considerable effort has been devoted at Area and District level to developing plans for services for the 'cinderella' groups. Health care planning teams, which operate at District level and involve the family doctor and social service staff as well as hospital staff, have collected information and made recommendations to District Management Teams. When working well, these have provided a basis for developing a coherent strategy for future development, and some health care planning teams have included members of CHCs in their discussions. They have also been an important aspect of collaboration between those administering and those providing health and social services.

Collaboration between health and social services

Co-ordination of health and social service policies and co-operation between staffs has remained a major issue since reorganisation, and it is, of course, linked to the development of community care. The 1974 reorganisation had one major weakness in relation to collaboration and that was the fact that the general practitioner remained outside the management and administrative structure of the NHS, although one of the three medical members of the District Management Team is in fact a GP. The GPs provide services under contract to the NHS and these contracts are managed by the Family Practitioner Committees which cover the same geographical areas as the AHAs. General practitioners value the independence which derives from the type of contract they have and remain, essentially, self-employed professionals who choose their own pattern and place of work, and yet they are the first point of contact for medical problems – and for many social problems, too – as far as the patient is concerned. GPs are an essential link in ensuring continuity of care between hospital and home. It can be difficult to slot them into the NHS structure as they have been educated professionally in a tradition of individual responsibility for patients which sometimes makes it difficult for them to work in a team except as leader (Dingwall 1980).

Perhaps one of the greatest stumbling blocks to continuity of care as well as to collaboration is this independent contractor status of the GP. Not only do individual practice arrangements vary greatly, but GP catchment areas for patients have no relationship to AHA or local government boundaries, although this does, however, widen the freedom of choice for both doctor and patient. The method of payment of GPs is based on different principles and their timetables and the organisation of their work are at variance with those of other professional groups, as indeed they vary from practice to practice. One of the common criticisms of case conferences is the low level of attendance by GPs, but conferences are often held at times which clash with surgery hours and home visits. Only a fairly large practice can cover for a GP attending case conferences and committee meetings.

There have, of course, been changes in the pattern of general practice since the 1940's, in particular the move from single-handed general practice to group practices. Less rapid has been the growth of health centres which were encouraged by the 1946 Act and grew in number in the 1970's: there were 212 health centres in 1972 and well over 800 at the end of the decade. In health centres, and in many group practices, and indeed where GPs practise single-handed, health visitors and district nurses may be attached. Attachment is the administrative arrangement whereby health visitors, district nurses, midwives and, occasionally, social workers work together to provide services for all the patients who are registered with a particular general practitioner. Whilst enabling community nursing staff to have a closer and more effective relationship with the family doctor concerned, success does depend upon personalities rather than on any formal mechanism. Such factors as whether or not office space is allocated to health service staff can have an important effect upon the way time is spent at the practice premises. In fact, attachment tends to work better when operated from purpose-built health centres than from the more usual general practitioner's surgery. Increased communication between nursing staff and the GP is a major gain from attachment, but there is also a loss. The patients on a GP's list can be widely spread, and in urban areas there may be a considerable overlapping of practices. Apart from time spent visiting, the intimate knowledge gained when a health visitor knows a small area well (and is herself well known within it) is itself valuable in the early detection, and even the prevention, of problems. A survey carried out in 1974 showed that 68% of practices had attached nurses (Royal Commission 1979). The trend, together with the increase of professional self-confidence of nurses in the community, has helped to develop the concept of the primary health care team. This rests on the idea of a number of health workers working together for a common purpose. One GP describes it as the 'delegation of responsibility to health visitors, district nurses, practice nurses and social workers. The GP sits in the middle like a spider in his web' (Dingwall 1980). Other observers see the relationship as one of equal partnership between different professionals.

There is a great deal of referral to social services departments from the health services: Goldberg (1977) found that 21% of referrals to a social services area office came from medical or health service staff. Collaborative co-ordination may also occur at the strategic planning level through the Joint Consultative Committees set up under the 1974 reorganisation.

Joint Consultative Committees

Joint Consultative Committees were set up as part of the reorganisation of 1974 to help to co-ordinate local authority provision of social services, housing, education and environmental health services with the provision of health services. The Committees consist of representatives of the relevant local authority committees and of the AHA. Their functioning is clearly of great importance in planning the provision of social, health and other relevant services (eg. sheltered housing, special schools) for particular client groups. To encourage joint planning, a system of *joint financing* was introduced in 1976. Under this system, local authority schemes which can be shown to save the NHS money can receive NHS money to pay for 60% of the capital cost of a project, and part of the running costs for a limited period. Projects financed in this way include hostels for the mentally handicapped, the development of a night sitting service — even a new lift in a residential home for the elderly might be included, on the grounds that more dependent residents can be kept for a longer time in the community, thus delaying their demand for a hospital bed. It could be argued that joint financing, simply because money is involved, is a more important way of bringing social service and health service planning together than the Joint Consultative Committee structure alone.

Joint Care Planning Teams

In addition to joint financing, Health Care Planning Teams also bring together officers from the Health District and those from local authorities. In some health districts these joint care planning teams include representatives from community health councils. Health care planning teams focus on particular groups or needs in the community, eg. mentally handicapped people or family planning services. In addition, the more complex structure of the NHS planning system requires plans to be passed from District to Area, and from Area to Region; this system has been criticised for causing unnecessary delay and uncertainty (Sargeant 1979).

It is the complexity of this planning system which brought criticism from the Royal Commission, reflected in *Patients First*. The system undoubtedly is complex and unwieldly and, particularly at joint consultative committee level, its value is doubtful. Each side (NHS and local authority) tends to follow its own organisational goals, viewed from its own perspective, reporting its plans to the 'other side' rather than planning complementary services. However, no real evaluation has been undertaken on the benefits of the collaborative aspect of the planning system within the NHS.

Little is known – perhaps surprisingly – about the extent to which care in the community actually has developed. The Royal Commission attempted to answer this question, but found information difficult to obtain. Although out-patient care had increased relative to in-patient care, and despite an increase in the numbers of the elderly, the numbers of patients in geriatric departments has remained constant. The numbers of nurses employed in the community, however, show the same levels of increase, overall, as those of hospital staffs between 1974 and 1977 (Royal Commission 1979).

Industrial relations in the NHS

If resource allocation and the slow move towards an increasing emphasis on community care has been one important issue in the NHS in the 1970's, industrial relations has been another which is at least as important. The work-force in the NHS is large and highly stratified, with workers having very different levels of pay, status and power over their own work situation. At the top of the hierarchy are the consultants and senior administrators who are part of a larger group of doctors and administrators. Nurses (over 400,000 of them) are the largest group in the NHS workforce. Unskilled and semi-skilled ancilliary workers are the next largest group at 200,000.

Industrial action to improve pay and conditions of service has been taken by virtually every group of workers within the NHS – increasingly so in the 1970's. The reasons for the changing industrial relations are complex. The level of inflation and financial restraint is one part of the explanation; another is the increasing specialisation and division of labour within the NHS, which makes chains of control and command longer and more complex and affects roles and relationships in the actual work setting. Industrial relations tended to be managed informally before the 1974 reorganisation, but since then work roles and relationships have changed. Yet channels of communication have not always improved – and sometimes have never been established. The NHS is very large and also very young: it is not surprising that it is facing these problems. The increasing role of trade unionism, which affects all NHS staff from consultants to the newest member of the domestic staff, is relevant to this discussion, but its relevance to nurses is discussed in Chapter 9.

The consumer and the NHS

Just as the growth of trade unionism is relevant to a discussion of the NHS so is the growth of consumerism. The 1970's has been a period during which patients' views and experiences of the NHS have been of more concern to policy makers, and patients have been more ready to give their views.

The Royal Commission commissioned a special survey on this issue, and found, as previous surveys of this kind had found, a very high level of satisfaction with the NHS among its users. Critics have argued that the increasing size of hospitals, ever more complex technologies and the larger bureacracy create organisations which exist for themselves rather than for the patient. It is futher argued that, apart from Community Health Councils (whose very existence was challenged in *Patients First*), health authorities are not sufficiently responsive to the consumer, or to representatives of his interests. Complaints systems are inadequate and not widely publicised, and quality controls are hard to identify. A variety of ways of protecting the patient do, in fact, exist, but how adequate are they in practice? The mechanisms available include the Health Advisory Service and the various complaints procedures.

The Health Advisory Service (HAS, formerly the Hospital Advisory Service) was set up following publication in 1969 of the Report of the Committee of Enquiry into Conditions at Ely Hospital. (It should be noted that this Enquiry was instituted only after disturbing stories about the hospital had appeared in the popular press.) The Health Advisory Service reports directly to the Secretary of State for Health and Social Services, and its function is to help to improve the management of patient care in individual hospitals (and in the community health services) by constructive criticism and by spreading knowledge of good practices and good ideas. It also advises the Secretary of State on the condition of hospitals and community health facilities, which it does through the medium of its annual reports, concentrating on disadvantaged groups such as the elderly, the mentally disordered, the disabled and the mentally handicapped.

The HAS operates by sending a multi-disciplinary team (consisting of a doctor, a nurse, an administrator, etc) to visit a hospital or other health care agency. The visit may last for several days, during which the members of the team will talk to most of the hospital's staff and take a detailed look at the quality of the health care being provided. The team then compiles a report which is sent to the Secretary of State and to the institution visited. The report and its implications and recommendations are discussed by senior staff of the hospital or agency concerned, and also by the team and staff at the DHSS. The membership of the teams is changed frequently to ensure that the participants are actively in touch with current practice and suitably experienced in the specialities of the service whose work is being surveyed.

The effectiveness of the HAS is limited, as it has no real power to see that its recommendations are implemented. Normansfield Hospital (for the mentally subnormal) had been visited well before the Enquiry which reported in 1978 had been set up; there had also been a number of similar Enquiries in addition to that at Ely (1969)—

Farleigh (1971), Whittingham (1972) – and Normansfield is only the most recent. Perhaps the Normansfield Report is the most depressing, as it showed that although the responsible authorities had known about and reported on the adverse conditions that had existed at the hospital since 1970 nothing had been done to change the management structure (Klein 1979).

Complaints

Complaints against family practitioners, dentists, pharmacists and ophthalmic practitioners, ie. those professionals providing services under contract to the Family Practitioner Committee (FPC), are made by the complainant to the FPC, which organises special Service Committees to hear them.

In the case of the services managed by an AHA, the AHA itself is responsible for its own enquiries, despite the Davies Committee's recommendation that a standard procedure be introduced (DHSS 1973). Public enquiries may be set up by the Secretary of State to investigate particular allegations – as happened with the mental handicap hospitals already mentioned.

Complaints may also be channelled through MPs who may ask questions in Parliament or write to the Minister. Members of the public may also write directly to the Minister involved. MPs and local councillors usually hold regular surgeries where they hear complaints and generally help their constitutents.

Since 1974, a Parliamentary Commissioner for the Health Services (there is also one for local government) has dealt with complaints from individuals. The Health Services Commissioner can, however, only deal with complaints after they have been made to the appropriate health authority. If the explanation is still not satisfactory to the complainant, the Commissioner may take up the complaint. He has no jurisdiction over matters relating to *clinical* judgement (and this also applies to the complaints procedure operated by the FPC), but this point is currently under discussion. The Commissioner publishes annual reports, and that for 1978–79 examined a large number of complaints relating to the care of the elderly in hospital. Although care which involves a medical judgement does not come under the jurisdiction of the Commissioner, nursing care does and in his annual reports the Commissioner often discusses cases in which the relatives of the patient were distressed by what they considered to be inadequate standards of nursing care.

Community Health Councils help to give the consumer a voice in the running of the health service, and may help patients to make their complaints effectively, although the CHCs often minimise the importance of the latter role. Some CHCs have collected information on the health care needs of special groups, including ethnic minorities, have undertaken research into locally-provided maternity services, and documented the cumulative effect of bed closures in the London area. However, they have often been ignored in the period of rapid cuts in planned public expenditure, and a way round the obligation to consult CHCs over, for example, bed closures has been found (ie. calling the closure 'temporary'). Nevertheless, for the individual with a complaint the CHC Secretary is able, through knowledge of the health service procedures and ability to present the material of the complaint clearly, to offer positive help. This role in helping complainants may well partly explain the hostility towards CHCs often found amongst professional and administrative NHS staff.

Last, but by no means least, especially in terms of finance, the consumer may turn to the civil courts if dissatisfied with the level of medical care provided, and if negligence can be shown to have occurred.

Patients First: the structure for the 1980s?

The end of perhaps the most turbulent decade in the history of the NHS has brought yet another proposal for restructuring – the consultative document *Patients First* (DHSS 1979), and a Circular from the DHSS, *Health Service Development: Structure and Management*, was sent out in 1980. The new decade began, in fact, with the presentation to Parliament of a Health Services Bill which would enable the changes proposed in *Patients First* to be implemented.

In many ways the proposals are a retreat from the 1974 structure. The major criticism of the 1974 reorganisation made in *Patients First* is about the management and planning structure '... the machinery for decision making is expensive, cumbersome and slow.

Matters which could be corrected in minutes or hours now take months with the obvious effect of slowing down the whole service'.

The Royal Commission (1979) had suggested that the health services could be seen in terms of two main functions: (a) the planning of services and (b) the delivery of these to the patient. *Patients First* follows this reasoning. The document recommends that the AHAs should be abolished, that management should be strengthened at district level, which is the point of delivery of services to the patient. Planning would take place at two levels only: region and district. Thus, new District Health Authorities (DHAs) would replace AHAs.

In some areas the new authorities are likely to cover the same areas as the existing districts, and in others, they would be formed by a merging of two or more districts. Implicit in these proposals is a move away from centralisation: the new authorities should '. . . feel themselves responsible for meeting local needs' (*Patients First* 1979).

The new DHAs are likely to include 16 members appointed by the RHA to include four members representing local authorities whose role would be to reflect local needs, as well as two doctors (a hospital consultant and a GP), a nurse a university member and a trade unionist. The idea of consensus management by senior administrative, nursing and medical staff in hospital and community services is retained. However, greater emphasis is given to the need for individual responsibility for sector management, so that responsibility lies with individuals as well as the 'management'.

In the short space of five years, notions of what is 'good' for the health service have changed. What will go and what will be retained? The stress on the importance of common boundaries between health and social services in local authorities has been dropped. The new health authorities will not necessarily be co-terminous with local authorities, and although the importance of collaboration is still stressed it will now depend on professional motivation.

The Joint Consultative Committee structure will remain, but the complicated planning machinery will be drastically reduced. The role of the Regions is, therefore, unlikely to grow as some services, such as specialist care for the mentally handicapped, which must be provided across larger areas than those of health districts, are likely to be provided by one DHA on behalf of another. Also under threat in the consultative paper are the Community Health Councils.

It is the cost of the CHCs which concerns the Conservative government – £4m in 1979/80 (*Patients First* 1979) – and it is ironic that a document entitled *Patients First* should suggest abolishing the consumer's role in the NHS.

The Royal Commission argued that '. . . CHCs have made an important contribution towards ensuring that local opinion is represented in health service management. They need additional resources to fulfil this task more effectively'. On the other hand, *Patients First* suggests that the need for separate consumer representation is less clear when members of the DHA will be 'less remote' from local services. However, members of the DHA will be appointed by the regions, and it is difficult to see how they could be said to 'represent' the consumer, when there are no formal channels for interaction, and this responsibility is not spelt out.

Gone too is the stress, given in pre-1974 thinking and White Papers, on the importance of developing community health services and countering the dominance of the hospital in patient care. The consultative paper, by defining the operational unit as 'a hospital and its associated community services', is likely to strengthen the claims of hospitals to resources, particularly as they may be encouraged to raise finances from outside the NHS.

Family Practitioner Committees are to remain as they are, contrary to the Royal Commission's recommendations, again a sign that the attempt to plan for integrated patient care has been abandoned. The message of *Patients First* and the Circular that followed it is clear: minimum change at minimum cost, with political conflicts over resource allocation removed to a less visible level of government, or regional, level. And the challenge to the NHS of the consumer view, as put forward by CHCs, was under threat until late in 1980, when their continuance was accepted by the government.

No matter what changes eventually result from the process of consultation following publication of *Patients First*, the experience of reorganisation has forced all who work in the health services, particularly those involved in any form of management, to learn new ways of working together, and to gain experience in determining priorities (individually and collectively).

The new DHAs will have greater power to determine their own

organisation and manning levels. Superficially, the DHAs may look a little like a return to the pre-1974 Hospital Management Committees. The analogy is false. The economic, political and social environment of health care has radically changed. What must never be forgotten is that the NHS is the biggest organisation in the world (Brown 1979). It is not a profit-making organisation but one concerned with care to the patient. It is also a relatively young service which must experiment in different ways of caring. If the reorganisation of 1974 has made those working in the NHS more flexible and adaptive to change, then it will have taught a valuable lesson.

Policy making in the health service

This account of the NHS has implicitly suggested that governments have the major role in initiating new policy and in effecting policy implementation through overall public expenditure control. Governments also react to demands for policies both from within and outside Parliament and must also rely on the informal support of the pressure groups, professional groups and trade unions.

Behind the rules, both formal and informal, which regulate relationships between groups, inside and outside government, lie general understandings which can be stretched, negotiated, argued about – as well as ignored at convenient moments. One of the great difficulties facing any minister is that of reconciling the role of employer of a large labour force with the role of provider of a service without direct charge to the public. Any policy being promoted for the public must also seek to accommodate the workforce: hence the emphasis on the negotiations with the various interest groups involved.

Since the 1960's, with the emphasis on planning, management and public expenditure control, much more monitoring and guidance from the top downwards has been taking place in the health services; this has increased the amount of conflict (eg. RAWP). This factor has combined with sharply reduced growth in public sector spending, compared to the inflation rate, and has affected some interest groups more than others; for example, London teaching hospitals may feel deprived, but less so than inner city Districts which feel that the London teaching hospitals are taking too many resources.

Conflict has also increased as various occupational groups within the hospital service have withdrawn their labour in the process of negotiating wages and conditions of service. In a highly inter-dependent workforce this causes highly-publicised breakdowns in the care of patients. Conflicts such as these place great strain on all who work in the NHS. Conflict has increased, also, perhaps, because of the proliferation of professional organisations – for example, medicine continues to sub-divide, each sub-division forming an interest group. The same happens in other skilled and unskilled branches of hospital work.

It is also important to remember that the way in which this book has looked at the health and social services has been with a *pluralist* view. This means it has been assumed that the political systems within the NHS can manage such conflict, and that power within the health service is very widely shared. As a result of these factors, change is slow and piecemeal, and policy modification is a result of bargaining between equally powerful goups. Many writers have argued that this is not true within the NHS, as the medical profession have more power than other groups, achieved through the network of inter-connecting committees and pressure groups active within, and in relation to, the DHSS. Their power also comes from a specialised area of knowledge which historically has dominated the health services. Changes occur, according to this analysis, only when groups within the medical profession see advantages in such changes, ie. doctors are seen as the major political influence.

Another criticism of the *pluralist* model accepted here comes from the *social class* model of the health services, and this perspective is one that sees an economically dominant class in Britain. This social class is further seen as exercising decisive economic and political power. This view, put forward by Navarro (1978), suggests that the health service represents a class interest, that the economy needs an active workforce, and stresses the extent of inequalities in health care provision. Allied to this, is the view that the NHS faces the problem of handling the anomaly that profits are made from anti-health activities (eg. selling tobacco and alcohol). The health of the economy is measured by factors such as growth in the rate of car sales, but the NHS has to deal with the expensive results of road accidents and the effects of atmospheric pollution.

Whichever view is taken of the dominant interests in policy making in the NHS, there is no doubt that such conflicts are now more visible and widely debated. It may be that this is all part of the shift in the definition of priorities in the care and treatment of health and illness, outlined at the very beginning of this chapter. These conflicts are likely at least to simmer over the next decade. The structural changes proposed for the 1980's may serve to contain the conflicts as the delivery of services takes precedence over attempts to make that delivery more equal between different areas, and district managements have more responsibility for reducing and resolving conflict in their own 'territory'.

As the emphasis on planning for *future* delivery of services takes a less central part, the quality of care and the co-ordination and continuity of care will depend more on the efforts of staff at the grass-roots level – the nurses, doctors and social workers who work in the community. Much will depend on their ability to work out ways of solving the problems they encounter in the face of social and demographic changes which are likely to lead to heavier demand and higher expectations in a period of virtually nil growth for the NHS.

References

Abrams P. (1977) Community Care: Some Research Problems and Priorities. *Policy and Policies*, V. 6 (2)

Beveridge W. (1942) *Social Insurance and Allied Services*. Cmd 6404. London: HMSO

Brown R. G. S. (1979) *Reorganising the National Health Service: A Case Study in Administrative Change*. Oxford: Blackwell & Robertson

Carrier J. (1978) Positive discrimination in the allocation of NHS resources. In M. Brown & S. Baldwin (eds) *The Yearbook of Social Policy 1977*. London: Routledge and Kegan Paul

Chester T. E. (1979) A better way to pay for health care? An essay in comparative analysis. *National Westminster Bank Quarterly Review*, Nov

Crossman R. H. S. (1972) *A Politician's View of Health Service Planning: 13th. Maurice Block Lecture*. University of Glasgow

Dingwall R. (1980) Problems of teamwork in primary care. In Lonsdale S., Webb A. & Briggs T. L. (eds) *Teamwork in the*

Personal Social Services and Health Care. London: Croom Helm

DHSS (1973) *Report of the Committee on Hospital Complaints Procedures* (Chairman: Sir M. Davies) London: HMSO

DHSS (1976) *Fit for the Future. Report of the Committee on Child Health Services* (Chairman: Professor D. Court). Cmnd 6684. London: HMSO

DHSS (1976) *Prevention and Health Everybody's Business: A Reassessment of Public and Personal Health.* London: HMSO

DHSS (1976) *Priorities for Health and Personal Social Services in England: A Consultative Document.* London: HMSO

DHSS (1976) *Sharing Resources for Health in England: A Report of the Resources Allocation Working Party.* London: HMSO

DHSS (1977) *Priorities in the Health and Social Services: The Way Forward.* London: HMSO

DHSS (1978) *Collaboration in Community Care: A Discussion Document.* London: HMSO

DHSS (1979) *Patients First: A Consultative Paper on the Structure and Management of the NHS in England and Wales.* London: HMSO

DHSS (1980) *Health Service Development: Structure and Management* HC(80)8 LAC(80)3. London: HMSO

Goldberg M. (1977) Towards accountability in social work. *British Journal of Social Work*, **7**(3)

Harbridge E. (1980) Co-operation: the right bricks for the job. *Community Care*, 13 March

Hart J. T. (1971) The inverse care law. *Lancet*, i, 405–412

Illsley R. (1976) *Health and Health Policy: Priorities for Research*, London: Social Science Research Council

Klein R. (1978) Normansfield: vacuum of management in the NHS. *British Medical Journal*, **2**, 1802–1804

Levitt R. (1976) *The Reorganised National Health Service.* London: Croom Helm

Mackenzie W. J. M. (1979) *Power and Responsibility in Health Care: the NHS as a Political Institution.* Oxford University Press

McKeown T. (1978) *The Role of Medicine: Dream, Mirage or Nemesis.* Oxford: Basil Blackwell

Ministry of Health (1920) *Consultative Council on Medical and Allied Services Interim Report.* (Chairman: Sir B. Dawson) London: HMSO

Ministry of Health (1962) *A Hospital Plan for England and Wales.* Cmnd 1604. London: HMSO

Ministry of Health (1963) *Health and Welfare: the Development of Community Care Plans for the Health and Welfare Services of Local Authorities in England and Wales.* London: HMSO

Morris P. (1969) *Put Away: A Sociological Study of Institutions for the Mentally Retarded.* London: Routledge & Kegan Paul

Navarro V. (1978) *Class Struggle, the State and Medicine: An Historical and Contemporary Analysis of the Medical Sector in Great Britain.* England: Martin Robertson

Office of Health Economics (1979) *Compendium of Statistics.* London: Office of Health Economics

Owen D. (1976) *In Sickness and in Health: the Politics of Medicine.* London: Quartet Books

Porritt A. (1962) *A Review of the Medical Services in Great Britain.* London: Medical Services Review Committee Social Assay

Report of the Health Service Commissioner (1978/9). London: HMSO

Report of the Committee of Enquiry into Allegations of Ill-treatment of Patients and Other Irregularities at Ely Hospital, Cardiff. (1969) Cmnd 3975. London: HMSO

Report of the Farleigh Hospital Committee of Enquiry. (1971) Cmnd 4557. London: HMSO

Report of the Committee of Enquiry into Whittingham Hospital (1972) Cmnd 4861. London: HMSO

Report of the Committee of Enquiry into Normansfield Hospital (1978) Cmnd 7357. London: HMSO

Robb B. (1967) *Sans Everything: A Case to Answer.* London: Nelson

Royal Commission on the Law Relating to Mental Illness and Mental Deficiency, 1954–1957 (1959) *Report.* Cmnd 169. London: HMSO

Royal Commission on the National Health Service (Chairman: Sir Alec Merrison) (1979) *Report.* Cmnd 7615. London: HMSO

Sargeant T. (1979) Joint care planning in the health and personal social services. In Booth T. A. (ed) *Welfare, Social Policy and the Expenditure Process.* England: Martin Robertson

Taylor J. (1979) Hidden labour and the National Health Service. In Atkinson P., Dingwall R. & Murcott A. (eds) *Prospects for the National Health Service*. London: Croom Helm

Titmuss R. (1970) *The Gift Relationship: From Human Blood to Social Policy*. London: Allen & Unwin

Townsend P. (1964) *The Last Refuge: A Survey of Residential Institutions and Homes for the Aged in England and Wales*. London: Routledge & Kegan Paul

Watkin B. (1978) *The National Health Service: the First Phase 1948–1974 and After*. London: Allen & Unwin

Chapter 7

The Personal Social Services

Judith Allsop

Introduction – the structure of the Social Services Departments

Social Services Departments (SSDs) were established in 1970, following the recommendations of the Seebohm Committee (Seebohm Report 1968) that 'A community-based and family-orientated service available to all' should be provided by local authorities through social service departments. Services which had been previously provided by a number of local authority departments were amalgamated into one department, headed by a Director of Social Services. The Director was made responsible to a Social Services Committee composed of elected local councillors. The 1970 Act established a department with broad functions for a wide range of client groups, with an emphasis on the accessibility of these services to the public. From 1974, following local government reorganisation, the services were provided in England by non-metropolitan counties, metropolitan districts, and London boroughs.

Social services departments have become large and complex organisations, providing a wide and varied range of services, mostly in kind, but sometimes in cash, to individuals and their families. Through at least 15 Acts of Parliament SSDs are able to provide residential accommodation, meals on wheels, and home helps; they supervise child minding and provide transport and recreational activities. They also provide supplementary services such as adaptations to the home, help with telephones, mobility training and sheltered employment and day centres. These services are aimed primarily at children in need and their families, the elderly, the physically ill and physically handicapped, the mentally ill and mentally handicapped and children whose needs become obvious through Juvenile Court proceedings. At the discretion of the local authority, groups such as the single homeless, battered wives, and alcoholics may be helped. Services are provided in a variety of different settings. Social work support, the home help service and meals on wheels operate in people's own homes; day care services are provided for the elderly and the mentally handicapped, and the residential institutions provided include homes for the elderly, hostels for the mentally ill and community homes for children deprived of a normal home life or at risk. Figure 7.1 shows the scope of social service departments, both in terms of objectives and of activity undertaken.

These services are carried out by a large administrative structure, centrally based, as the provision of services must be planned and coordinated. Services may also be provided through voluntary agencies such as Citizens' Advice Bureaux, local branches of Family Service Units or Age Concern. SSDs are also responsible for the registration and inspection of some services provided through the private sector, for example, child minders and profit-making homes for the elderly.

Most SSDs have a research section, which is concerned with collecting basic information on needs in the area, and considering alternative policies. A major task of the higher management staff of SSDs has become the promotion of collaboration between SSDs and health services, as well as between SSDs and other departments concerned with those in need, such as education and housing departments. Liaison with social security offices is also an important aspect of the work of social services departments, as poverty lies behind so many of the problems of the department's clients.

Next to education departments and housing, social services departments are the biggest spenders in local government, and in 1975 the personal social services in the UK consumed 1.9% of all public expenditure, or about £1,000m. Nearly half of this was spent on residential care, and the largest group receiving this service was the elderly (followed by children). In terms of staffing, the elderly were again shown to be the major users of resources, as they received a major share of domiciliary services, especially the home help service, as well as residential care. Field social workers (professional trained social workers), and also social work assistants (who are untrained) or trainees (who plan to take a professional qualification), made up only 9% of the total staff of SSDs in the com-

OBJECTIVES AND ACTIVITIES
OF SOCIAL SERVICE DEPARTMENTS

GENERAL OBJECTIVE	SPECIFIC OBJECTIVE	ACTIVITY
Support and maintenance of family	To relieve families in stress: to keep children with their parents: to prevent loss of home	Personal help, and information; cash or material aid; domestic help (e.g. home help, laundry service); removal of member of family during day or for short period (e.g. holiday) or long period (residential care)
Support and strengthening of handicapped individuals	To help people manage their handicap	Personal help, advice and information; aids and adaptations in the home; mobility training for blind
	To provide occupational, social and recreational activity for those excluded from 'normal' activities	Transport: occupational day centres; social day centres; luncheon clubs; holidays; entertainment (e.g. television, outings)
	To enable people to live in the community	Personal help, advice and information; domestic help; meals; aids and adaptations to housing
Provision of care for dependent individual without family	To provide a home	Residential care
	To provide a substitute family	Adoption; fostering; boarding-out schemes for adults
	To enable people to live in the community	Personal help, advice and information
Protection of vulnerable individuals	To prevent and deal with child abuse	Personal help to families; investigation of children 'at risk'; removal of child to substitute home
	To 'police' standards of care in the private sector	Registration, inspection and supervision of child-minders, private nurseries and playgroups; inspection and supvervision of private nursing homes etc.; protection of private foster children
Provision of social help in treatment of deviance	To help disturbed or 'deviant' children and adults	Personal help, advice and information; intermediate treatment; rehabilitation for adults; residential care
Strengthening the community	To promote activities and action benefiting the community as a whole	Community work e.g. encouragement of tenants' associations; holiday projects; playgroups

Fig 7.1 From McCreadie C. *The Personal Social Services*. Policy Studies Institute 1977. Reproduced by kind permission of the author and of the Institute

munity in 1975 (Personal Social Services Council 1977). This group, although a small proportion of total staff, are the most visible group of social service employees (visible to the public and the media). They make up the social work teams which are based on area offices spread through each local authority. Social workers may be the channel through which other services are obtained, eg. home helps or meals on wheels, a place in a day centre or a bed in a residential home. In this way, part of their task is analogous to that of general practitioners or health visitors, who also mobilise services for their patients.

The Seebohm Committee's intention was to make SSDs readily available to the public, which is why it recommended the establishment of area offices, each to serve some 50,000 people. Social work teams would operate from area offices, and carry a mixed case load of clients. Prior to 1970 social work had developed into a number of specialist branches, linked to the fragmented administrative development of social services. Children's departments employed social workers who had been trained as child care officers; mental health sections of the local health authority would employ psychiatric social workers; hospitals would employ medical social workers; welfare departments would have specialists working with the blind and the deaf . . . and so on. By the 1960's the new Certificate in Social Work courses were producing social workers with a more flexible approach but their work-load was determined by their setting. Following the Seebohm Report there was a move towards a more general training of social workers, supervised by the newly-formed Central Council for Training and Education in Social Work. It was hoped that the social work team, if not every social worker in it, would be able to work with a wide range of clients, but specialist advisers for particular client groups (eg. the mentally ill, the blind) were appointed usually to work with the SSD itself, not with any area-based team. Hospital-based social workers are still employed by SSDs despite their hospital setting. The major division now between types of social work skills is between methods of work rather than client groups: case work, group work and community work techniques.

In terms of overall expenditure and provision of services, the 1970's were a period of rapid growth for the personal social services. In 1968, the share of public expenditure attributable to these services was 0·8% and by 1975 this had risen to 1·9% – a faster growth than the other social services. Between 1965 and 1975 actual expenditure on health services and on education quadrupled, but spending on the personal social services increased ten-fold. However, it must be remembered that they began from a very low base: in 1975 for every £5 spent on health and £6.50 on education, only £1 was spent on the personal social services (McCreadie 1977).

This increase in spending hides very important differences *between* local authorities (as shown in the DHSS's Social Service Statistics for 1976) despite DHSS attempts to encourage SSDs to provide a minimum level of service, measured, for example, by the number of home helps per 10,000 people aged over 65 years. In 1976/7, to give another example, spending on aids for the disabled varied from £453 per 1,000 of the population in Wakefield, to £5 in Knowsley (Ashley 1980).

The rapid growth of services has had benefits and disadvantages for those working in the social services. Certainly, career opportunities, salary and promotion prospects increased, as was intended by the Seebohm Committee, but there have been costs. These are discussed by Parsloe & Stevenson in their study of social service teams (DHSS 1978). Because of the broad range of services they provide, SSDs receive a wide range of demands and requests. One social worker quoted in their study said ' . . . there seems to be no clear-cut jurisdiction for this department. Probation officers (who are social workers in the court) have their own clientele, they know when people come under their umbrella and when they don't. A generic department doesn't know. The social services department is the department everyone else sends people to'. Added to this there is a potentially infinite demand for social services, and social workers are therefore faced with the necessity of deciding between priorities, often against the background of a lack of clarity over objectives and roles. In the 1980's, as the public expenditure cuts bite, decisions of this kind will become more frequent.

The growth of expenditure on personal social services has been due not only to the establishment of SSDs but also to structural changes in society which similarly effect health service provision. Of these changes, the ageing population is particularly important. The changes in the population structure, caused partly by the falling birth and death rates, have been discussed in earlier chapters. The elderly are, however, not the only vulnerable group to increase in size. Families with single parents are more numerous, now, accounting for 10% of all families. Aspirations and expectations of the general public continue to rise, and this is sometimes expressed in new legislation (eg. the Chronically Sick and Disabled Act 1971) or in government reports (eg. Better Services for the Mentally Ill, DHSS 1975).

The services provided are based on a number of Acts of Parliament, the most important of which are discussed below.

Functions of the Social Service Departments

Under Part III of the National Assistance Act 1948 local authorities had to provide residential care for the elderly and handicapped, which is why such accommodation is still sometimes called 'Part III accommodation', although that Act was incorporated into the 1970 Act under which SSDs were formed. Also important for the elderly is the Health Services and Public Health Act 1968, which placed a duty upon local authorities to provide a home help service, and to promote the welfare of the elderly.

The Chronically Sick and Disabled Act 1970 made it mandatory for SSDs to estimate the numbers of physically handicapped in their areas, and to encourage registration. Registration implies an obligation to provide a wide range of services, (eg. personal aids to mobility, adaptations to property) – all services which aim to compensate for disability. Between March 1972 and March 1973 the number of disabled persons registered with SSDs doubled, from 300,000 to nearly 600,000. Despite this growth, services vary from one local authority to another and as the public expenditure cuts begin to affect the quantity of SSD work, the disabled are unlikely, despite the 1970 Act, to escape the adverse effects of the cuts.

The Children's Act 1948 gave responsibility for children in need of care and protection to the newly-formed Children's Department. The Children's Act 1963 and the Children and Young Persons Act 1969 increased the responsibilities for children which were taken over by SSDs under the Social Services Act 1970.

The 1963 Act encouraged preventive social work with families, aimed at preventing children from being received into care, and it enabled social workers to make small financial payments to families under Section I of the Act in order to achieve this aim.

The 1969 Act transferred the care of young people coming before the courts from the probation service to local authority social workers, and they became responsible for a new type of client (people needing control as well as care), new kinds of residential institutions and new kinds of 'treatment', eg. intermediate treatment. The purpose of the Act was to prevent 'labelling' of young offenders and to encourage care within the area where they lived. The problems were that SSDs were given no extra resources, and had neither the staff to care adequately for the children now allocated to them, nor the appropriate residential accommodation.

The Children's Act 1980 is designed to bring together a large number of separate Acts relating to the social needs of children.

There was no legislation to improve the standards of care of other client groups, but several government publications recommended measures to raise standards of care and increase the range of facilities available, especially in the community. These publications include *Better Services for the Mentally Handicapped* (DHSS 1971), *Better Services for the Mentally Ill* (DHSS 1975) and *A Happier Old Age* (1978). Other changes included the establishment of Area Review Committees in cases of non-accidental injury to children. These publications and developments were aimed at promoting discussion among the professions and the public about good practice, but no extra funds were earmarked for the achievement of the levels of service recommended. Vulnerable groups, such as the elderly, are obviously growing at a faster rate than public expenditure, with obvious implications for the quantity and quality of work of the SSDs.

The increasing number of professionals and administrators employed in providing care in the social services contains its own impetus to growth. Social work staffs operate within a framework of very broadly-worded statutory obligations and this is coupled with an open-ended number of permissive powers under which additional services could be provided. This combination of factors, in conjunction with increasing public demand, lies behind the continuing pressure for more resources.

In the period from the mid-1970's onwards, with the beginning of the attempts to *curb* and later *cut* the growth of public expenditure in general and of the social services in particular, there has been increased emphasis on using both health and social service resources more effectively and efficiently. Two aspects of care on which attention has been focused are the contribution which voluntary organisations could make in supplementing and complementing publicly-provided care, together with the potential contribution of the volunteer for unpaid caring within the community. More thought has been given to the best means of increasing collaboration between the health and social services, particularly as this relates to care in the community rather than institutions. Before considering the role of voluntary organisations and methods of collaboration, the idea of community care in social services is discussed.

Community care

It is easier to trace the development of the use of the term community care in policy statements than to arrive at any one clear definition of the concept. The term was used in the late 1950's to describe the changes favoured in the Mental Health Act 1959. This was based on the principle of a mental health service which took patients out of the large institution and placed them in the community. The then Minister of Health argued that this was not just a local authority matter, as hospitals also had a part to play, whilst the co-operation of the public was also needed if patients were to be accepted into the community. (The development of community care in health services is discussed in Chapter 6.)

In practical terms, community care in social services meant day care centres, adult training centres, hostels, group homes, sheltered housing and other agencies to complement the work previously undertaken within the hospital – complementing the important development of the community psychiatric nurse. During the 1960's and 1970's the policy of providing smaller-scale residential or day care facilities developed in relation to other groups such as the elderly or the mentally handicapped. Nevertheless, the shortage of community facilities, and the variations between areas, are no doubt obvious to readers working in the health and social services.

Michael Bayley in his book *Mental Handicap and Community Care* (1973) drew attention to the important distinction between care BY the community and care IN the community. He pointed out that many clients need 24-hour care which cannot be met by statutory or voluntary services alone but relies on the part played by relatives, friends and neighbours. He argues that this informal network is as important as, if not more important than, the formal one, and the burden on the caring relative can too easily be taken for granted by those seeking to keep the patient in the community at *all* costs. The reductions in public expenditure are likely to lengthen the waiting lists for residential care and reduce the amount of community support services. It could be argued that the family will be asked to accept a burden of care which could have adverse effects on the health of the whole family. Lay and non-specialist care tends to depend on the existence of social networks which are more likely to be based on ties of kinship, religion or ethnic group than of the locality. Some forms of care bridge the clear-cut division between professional and lay care (eg. home helps, community workers, hostel provision). Perhaps these combinations of types of care are most likely to develop when public resources are being cut back, and it for this reason that it is important to consider the contribution of voluntary organisations and volunteers to the provision of welfare.

Voluntary organisations and volunteers

It is difficult to define voluntary organisations precisely, as many carry out the same functions as statutory bodies (eg. providing residential care for children). Some are financed wholly from public funds (eg. Women's Royal Voluntary Service), and many have professionally-trained staff (eg. the Family Service Units). Perhaps their only common characteristic is their independence from state control and their freedom to make their own policy.

There is little comprehensive information on the contribution of voluntary organisations to the total provision of caring services. The Personal Social Services Council, disbanded in 1980, carried out a limited study in 1976 of the manpower and training resources of 44 such organisations in England and Wales (PSSC 1976). They found that these organisations employed a paid workforce equal to one sixth of the comparable workforce in SSDs (including field work, residential and day care), and that they were also responsible for organising a considerable number of volunteers. Certainly, voluntary organisations continue to play their traditional role of supplementing state care, particularly in the provision of leisure activities, and they provide about 20% of residential accommodation for the elderly and for the physically and mentally ill (DHSS 1977).

Voluntary organisations also play a role in welfare provision which public services *cannot* or *will not* play. They frequently pioneer new forms of care for particular groups, such as battered wives, which are later often taken over by statutory authorities. They continue to provide services for groups such as the homeless single person where the state takes virtually no responsibility. Much youth work and work with immigrants is undertaken by voluntary bodies.

Voluntary organisations have been developing in new ways since the Second World War. There are more co-ordinating organisations which seek to make the work of voluntary bodies in particular areas of care more effective. At the same time they may act as pressure groups on the government, and sources of information for the public: examples of this would include Local Councils of Social Service, and Age Concern. There are also other self-help and mutual-aid groups, such as Gingerbread for one parent families, and Alcoholics Anonymous. Other organisations, such as the Society of Compassionate Friends, help parents whose child has died.

One of the strengths of the voluntary sector is that it offers alternative sources of care, and this is one way of combating the monopoly of the state services. They also tap resources in terms of finance and labour which would not otherwise be available for caring activities. Nowhere is this more true than in the contribution made by the *volunteer* as opposed to the *voluntary organisation*.

Voluntary help can be given in two major forms: in the giving of labour, as a direct service such as visiting the elderly, or in the giving of money. The State cannot, and perhaps should not, meet all needs for social care, particularly within the community, and volunteer help is part of the humane society to which we aspire (Titmuss 1970). Yet recently, we have seen a search for better ways of organising and finding community resources. Statutory authorities have themselves set up organisations, as the Home Office has set up the Voluntary Service Unit. Volunteer Bureaux are being organised at local level and Voluntary Service Organisers are now found in most hospitals and some SSDs – all aiming at a more rational recruitment and deployment of the volunteer. In some schemes a form of payment is made to encourage 'good neighbours' to take on a regular commitment to people who, provided such help is available, are able to look after themselves at home. Most successful are those volunteer systems which involve some kind of exchange, eg. sharing the care of young children, keeping an eye on an elderly person who in turn then acts as a baby sitter, etc.

If, then, social care in the community is to be developed the contribution of both voluntary organisations and the volunteer, as part of the caring network, would seem to be vital. Yet there are difficulties. Rights to such services do not have the same status as rights to statutory services. The voluntary contribution can be variable and uncertain.

In areas where care is most needed – the inner city or the seaside town with a high proportion of elderly – it may be particularly difficult to recruit volunteers. Specialised, professional health and social services are unlikely to diminish in importance, and neither is the importance of collaboration between these two services in the planning and delivery of effective care in the community – and in institutions. Methods of increasing collaboration – and some of the difficulties – are discussed later in this chapter but, before this we examine some of the problems relating to policy making in local authorities, in order to explain why such collaboration may be difficult to achieve.

Influences on policy making within local authorities

Policy making in the personal social services therefore takes place in a very different political climate from policy making in the health services. There are elected local authorities standing between central government and those providing and receiving the services of social services departments: each local authority is in one sense a political system in miniature (Stanyer 1976).

Each social services department is politically controlled by a committee of elected local authority councillors, to which the Director of Social Services is responsible, and this committee decides policy on social service provision, usually on the recommendation of the Director. The policy will be influenced by the overall objectives of the majority party in the Council, and this is particularly so in relation to financial allocations, for just as central government departments have to work within budgets laid down by the Treasury and Cabinet, so local authority departments work within a budget. The amount of the budget is determined by the level at which the Council have decided to fix the local rate and the level of Rate Support Grant allocated by the government.

The allocation of resources within the SSD is the product of a continuous process of bargaining between the professionals, the administrators and the elected representatives. Judge (1979) describes how the responsibility lies with the social services committee, largely influenced by their Chief Officer working within the constraints imposed by the Finance Committee, which in turn is constrained by the resources decided by the relevant government departments who, in turn, are constrained by the Treasury and Cabinet decisions on public expenditure. There is, therefore, a *hierarchy of rationing decisions* which react one upon another since no subordinate level passively accepts the allocations made from above.

The Department of the Environment is the most powerful of the government departments. It influences local authority expenditure through its grants for current spending, as well as controlling capital expenditure. Other departments also control capital expenditure, eg. the Department of Education when schools are to be built.

The DHSS influence on local authorities is exerted partly through the provision of loan capital for projects in the social services, and more recently, through the limited amounts of money made available under the Joint Financing scheme already described in Chapter 6. In principle, the level of loans relates to the levels negotiated with the Treasury, and to policy objectives of the Department. 'Bids' are made by SSDs for loans for particular projects and these bids are usually listed in order of priority. The system leads to much continuing negotiation between local authorities and central government, the outcome of which is not always in line with stated priorities. Central government does not always take into account that local authorities' overall planning systems involve several departments, such as education and housing, nor do they take into account relationships with the health authorities. Local authorities tend to bid for more loans than they need, in order to ensure that some at least of their priorities are achieved (Judge 1979).

Within local authorities, personal social services must compete with other departments for resources – with education, leisure, housing and so on. These departments also provide tangible services to the community and are also affected by government policies. Another set of decisions about who gets what at the local authority level may depend on the existence of a corporate plan which attempts to set out a strategy for the provision of local services, relating one service to another.

Within the SSD, priorities are decided within the constraints of the departmental budget, in relation to existing services, to the priorities of the political party in power, as well as the views of professional and administrative staff.

Levels of service within the SSD will vary. For example, services for the mentally ill may be well-developed, whilst those for the physically handicapped lag behind. This may be due to pressure group activity, or the particular interest of the Chairman of the Social Service Committee, or of the Director of the SSD, or more objective factors. One would expect services for the elderly to be well-developed in a local authority with a higher than average proportion of citizens over 65.

Local authorities are very diverse in their characteristics (eg. population structure, employment opportunities, housing stress), so they have very different social problems. The difference between rural and urban local authorities is but one obvious example. Readers will no doubt be aware of these kinds of variations, just by observing their own locality. They will be equally aware of the differences that can occur within a local authority and reflect different levels of need: poorer families might be found in one particular estate, the elderly in particular streets.

The rationale for locally-elected councils rests on their identification with the local community. Yet the result is that social services offer very different levels of care. Different patterns of provision can mean that while one local authority delivers meals on wheels seven days a week, another will deliver only up to three times a week. Elderly people living in a street where the local authority boundary falls may find they receive more favourable treatment than their neighbours on the opposite side!

Collaboration between the health and social services

'Collaboration cannot be left to depend merely on common boundaries (between authorities providing health and personal social services). Services of mutual concern have to be identified and arrangements made between the authorities to plan, develop and operate them so that they satisfy mutual needs' (DHSS: National Health Service Reorganisation 1972).

The need to co-ordinate the policies of separate departments and agencies providing welfare and to encourage co-operation between personnel involved with the same individuals, families and social problems, has long dominated discussions about social welfare. It has been believed that lack of co-ordination and co-operation leads to costly duplication of services and to gaps and ineffective services which fail to meet needs adequately. With the development of policies favouring care *in* the community and the clear administrative divide between health and social services which followed the Social Services Act 1970, as well as health and local government reorganisation, there has been a more explicit central government commitment to encouraging strategies for collaboration. For example, a senior nurse is appointed at AHA level to be responsible for contact with SSDs and a senior social worker for Health Service Liaison. Specialists in community medicine act as advisers to local authorities (eg. with regard to physically and mentally handicapped children). Shrinking budgets have increased the *urgency* but not necessarily the *likelihood* of cooperation, which depends more on personal factors than on administrative arrangements.

This section considers health/social service collaboration although it is only one aspect of the social service scene. The Central Policy Review Staff's publication *A Joint Framework for Social Policies* (1975) stressed the need for collaboration at all levels between social services, including housing, education and social security, in relation to problems like poverty and inner city deprivation. This was so that more could become known about the causes of such problems and those policy interventions which were effective. Non-accidental injury to children is another area where the causal factors are complex and perhaps obscure. Collaboration between a number of agencies is needed if an effective diagnostic and preventive service is to develop, involving a good working relationship between general practitioner, social worker, health visitor, paediatrician and the medical and nursing staff of hospital accident and emergency departments.

In the last chapter, the activities of Health Care Planning Teams, District Planning Teams and Joint Consultative Committees were discussed. Although concerned primarily with planning future developments, they also provide a forum of discussion for local authority and health service personnel where common problems, priorities and strategies can be discussed, with advantages for both services.

Collaboration also involves, at the operational level, case conferences, referral procedures, team work, and liaison schemes.

Case conferences Case conferences, at which one specific case is discussed in detail by the professions involved – but rarely with the client present – vary in length and formality. Participation may be limited to one professional group but, more commonly, a case conference will be inter-professional: the meeting may be short, on the spur of the moment, or a session may be planned in advance, with a set agenda. Case conferences are regularly used in cases of non-accidental injury, and will include representatives of the health services (eg. paediatrician, health visitor), voluntary organisations (eg. National Society for the Prevention of Cruelty to Children or Family Service Units), the social services department, and perhaps the police, education and housing authorities (DHSS 1978). Participation by general practitioners is unfortunately uncommon, partly because they are reluctant to devote the necessary amount of time, partly because the timing often conflicts with their surgeries, and partly because their value may not be apparent. GPs rarely initiate case conferences and are often worried by the issue of confidentiality.

Referral Social problems and requests for help do not necessarily come directly to the professional or agency best able to deal with them. In principle, all professionals in contact with the public, in the helping and caring services, need to be aware of the range of services available in their area, and to be able to refer patients or clients to the most appropriate provider of services.

Family practitioners are frequently the first point of contact for the patient in the community, but their knowledge of the range of services available through social and community health services is limited. (Personal Social Services Council 1978). Where the GP works closely with attached health visitors (as discussed in Chapter 6), this organisational isolation is reduced. A few practices may have attached social workers but this is less well accepted by both professions than the attachment of nurses.

Teamwork Teamwork is a concept which has been much debated both in health services and in social services (Hunt 1979; Lonsdale, Webb & Briggs 1980).

The term teamwork can be used to describe the relationship which develops between a number of people working together on a regular basis, in an organised way, usually under a nominated leader, to deal with particular problems. Within the health and social services there are area social work teams, primary health care teams, district planning teams and many others. It is a fashionable concept, although it is impossible to estimate at this stage how widespread and effective teamwork really is. Attachment, which is an important aspect of teamwork, is discussed in Chapter 6.

The future of collaboration   Much collaborative work is clearly going on in different areas, but more needs to be known about which forms work best, and why. Organisations have their own particular ways of working – different lines of authority, different forms of communication, different ideas about priorities; these ways of working are not necessarily understood by other agencies and/or other professionals. For example, a social worker may be faced with a particular statutory obligation to act (eg. over the reception of a child into care, or the operation of the emergency procedures of the Mental Health Act 1959) which must take precedence over other cases. Hospitals operate a 24-hour day, seven days a week; there may be the need to discharge an elderly person over a weekend, as an acute bed is urgently needed. Social workers do not have access to the full range of domiciliary services at weekends – indeed, there may not even be a duty social worker available to deal with the newly discharged, vulnerable patient. The fact that nurses' training now contains community experience may be one important means of persuading hospitals to modify discharge procedures in the interests of the vulnerable!

These factors make both collaboration and community care difficult to achieve, although there are continuing attempts to ensure better working relationships and better planning. Different professional training and attitudes can lead to ignorance of respective roles and even to doubts about the competence of other agencies and services, and this difficulty is made worse when the boundaries of work are unclear, as can happen between health visiting and social work.

Reorganisation of a service or a high turnover of staff can break tenuous or even established lines of communication. Many misunderstandings are caused by the different value systems of different kinds of professionals: non-judgemental attitudes and non-directive methods are stressed in social work whereas doctors and nurses learn to make quick, usually unchallenged, decisions about the care and cure of the ill patient. One solution is the proposal that there should be more common elements in the education and training of the caring professions.

A further (and possibly the most important) stumbling block to collaboration between services is the pressure of work and shortage of resources, which has been, and is likely to be, a continuing feature of provision. The Priorities in Health and Welfare document (1976) placed the community nursing services high on the list of priorities, with a proposed growth rate of 6% a year, yet the reality, in a time of cuts, is that staff training seems a painless and quick way of cutting expenditure, so health visitor training actually dropped after the Priorities document was published. Similarly, it is increasingly difficult for untrained social workers to be seconded to attend training courses. In addition, the growing workload of the district nurse must cause concern: 15,000 community nurses visit about 3·3 million patients a year – such a workload can hardly favour the development of high quality care.

The tragedy is that a situation where limited resources have to be divided between competing claims creates the conditions for *rivalry* rather than *co-operation*. Each professional group or agency has its own idea of priorities, and when health services personnel are involved, in the 1980's, with yet another reorganisation of the NHS, the situation might well be worsened.

Nevertheless, much useful collaborative work IS taking place, particularly in relation to non-accidental injury, and is discussed in Maureen Lahiff's book *Hard-to-Help Families* (1981) which is published in the same series as this book.

The future of the personal social services

Although spared the upheaval of reorganisation which faces NHS staff, SSDs face a period of public expenditure cuts, where the most vulnerable will be most at risk. The public's expectations will be disappointed, and professional staff frustrated. In an article outlining the detailed implications of the cuts for Kent Count Council, the Director of Social Services Nicolas Stacey (1980) wrote 'If we could reduce our management and administrative overheads by 20%, and frankly in a reasonably well-run department I do not believe it is possible to do this and keep a complicated machine running smoothly, it would only save £460,000, a little over 15% of the savings required. The balance of £2.5m would have to come from closing homes, reducing the home help service and cutting back on social workers, etc. This is why councils like Kent are hoping to avoid having to cut social services by as much as central government is recommending. They are all too painfully aware that savings cannot be achieved merely by cutting bureaucracy'.

'Most of us share the Prime Minister's concern to 'cut it', but I do not see how it can be done without changing the present system. Bureaucracy is a by-product of bigness. It is fuelled by the immense complexity of getting anything done, often because of well-intentioned but restricting central government legislation. Local government is even more complicated and hamstrung than big business because, quite properly, it is publicly accountable and democratically controlled, which is inevitably slow, cumbersome and increasingly expensive. If the economy of the country cannot sustain the expenditure required by a large public sector, then we must look for new ways of dealing with old problems. We should also ask whether big, bureaucratic, hierarchical, highly-unionised, cumbersome and cautious local government machines are the best instruments for delivering social services when these need to be personal, fast-reacting, flexible and compassionate to be effective'.

From discussing the very real problems of the social services departments with their vulnerable clients, we turn to housing provisions, which are relevant to the lives of everyone of us – rich or poor, weak or strong.

References

Ashley J. (1980) Reported in *Community Care*, 24th Jan.
Bayley M. (1973) *Mental Handicap and Community Care: A Study of Mentally Handicapped People in Sheffield*. London: Routledge & Kegan Paul

Central Policy Review Staff (1975) *A Joint Framework for Social Policies*. London: HMSO

DHSS (1971) *Better Services for the Mentally Handicapped*. Cmnd 4683. London: HMSO

DHSS (1972) *National Health Service Reorganisation, England: White Paper*. Cmnd 5055. London: HMSO

DHSS (1975) *Better Services for the Mentally Ill*. Cmnd 6233. London: HMSO

DHSS (1976) *Priorities for the Health and Social Services in England: A Consultative Document*. London: HMSO

DHSS (1977) *Health and Personal Social Service Statistics for England for 1976*. London: HMSO

DHSS (1978) *Collaboration in Community Care: A Discussion Document*. London: HMSO

DHSS (1978) *A Happier Old Age: A Discussion Document on Elderly People in our Society*. London: HMSO

DHSS (1978) *Social Service Teams: A Practioner's View*. (A report of the Social Work Research Project directed by O. Stevenson & P. Parsloe). London: HMSO

Hunt M. (1979) Possibilities and problems of inter-disciplinary teamwork. In Marshall, Preston-Shoot & Wincott (eds) *Teamwork: For and Against*. British Association of Social Workers

Judge K. (1978) *Rationing Personal Social Services*. London: Heinemann

Lahiff M. (1981) *Hard-to-Help Families*. Aylesbury: HM+M Publishers

Lonsdale S., Webb A. & Briggs T. L. (1980) *Teamwork in the Personal Social Services and Health Care*. London: Croom Helm

McCreadie C. (1977) The personal social services. In R. Klein (ed) *Inflation and Priorities: Social Policy and Public Expenditure 1975*. London: Policy Studies Institute

Personal Social Services Council (1976) *Voluntary Social Services Manpower Resources*. London: PSSC

Personal Social Services Council (1977) *Personal Social Services: Basic Information* London: PSSC

Report of the Committee on Local Authority and Allied Personal Social Services (1968) (Seebohm Report) Cmnd 3703. London: HMSO

Stacey N. (1980) Cutting back: the grim dilemma facing Kent. *The Times*, 23 Jan.
Stanyer J. (1976) *Understanding Local Government*. London: Collins/Fontana

Chapter 8

Housing

Jean Gaffin

Introduction

The relationship between health and housing is strong, but complex. Housing can precipitate or perpetuate episodes of acute ill health, the link between damp housing and chest conditions being an obvious example. Inadequate housing can prolong time spent in hospital; for example, the baby who cannot be discharged to her parents' inadequate flat, or the elderly man who cannot cope with the stairs to his rented bed-sitting room. The work of the community nurse may well be frustrated if her patients are ill housed, and the health visitor faced with a family in inadequate housing will find it hard to concentrate on questions of toilet training or immunisation when the mother is on tranquilisers to help her cope with the lack of a bathroom and with a shared kitchen! And how can the community nurse help the elderly arthritic patient who is housebound only because she cannot negotiate the front steps? One solution may be to enquire whether the social services department will pay for a ramp so that she can get out. Or, the local housing department might be asked if a purpose-built one-bedroom flat is available, or the SSD might be approached to see if a unit of sheltered accommodation, with a warden, might be available. Any of these courses of action depends on a range of factors relating to the policy and resources of the local authority concerned, but equally relevant is the kind of housing now occupied; whether it is local authority rented, privately rented or owned by the patient. Local authority transfers and adaptation to local authority and owner-occupied homes are easier than when a private landlord is involved.

One way of considering the tangle of our housing system is to look separately at the three sectors of the housing market: owner occupation, privately rented and local authority accommodation. In contrast with social security, social service or health service provisions, where the State is virtually totally involved, the housing market is dominated by the private sector. Over half the population meet their own housing needs, using privately-owned institutions such as estate agents and building societies, although State intervention is crucial in that the tax relief on mortgage repayments represents a substantial subsidy to the house purchaser – a large proportion of the population which any political party would hesitate to alienate! The private tenant is a shrinking minority and the local authority tenant a slowly-growing group, as Figure 8.1 shows.

The privately-rented sector covers both furnished and unfur-

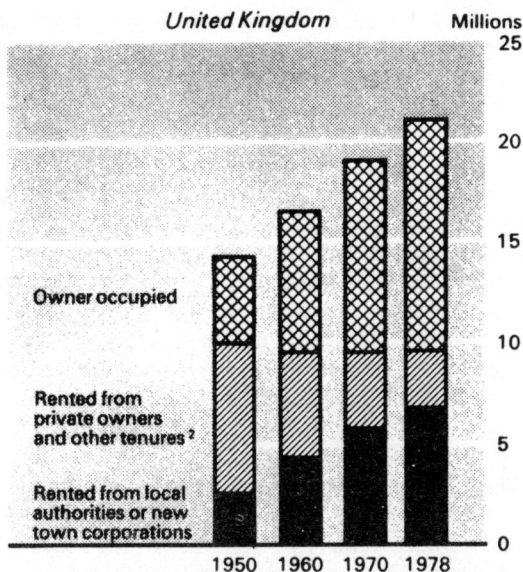

² Other tenures include dwellings rented with farms or business premises, and those occupied by virtue of employment.

Source: Housing and Construction Statistics, *Department of the Environment*

Fig 8.1 Stock of dwellings by tenure (from *Social Trends 10*, 1979. Reproduced by permission of the Controller of Her Majesty's Stationery Office)

nished property. Tenants vary widely, from the elderly couple renting part of a house, to the occupants of a large block of flats. Similarly, landlords vary – from the elderly widow whose husband bought a second house as an investment and source of income, to the large company which owns hundreds of properties. Conditions can vary from the dilapidated multi-occupied inner city house to the luxury of a Mayfair penthouse.

The balance between the landlord's desire for a fair return on his investment and the tenant's desire for adequate accommodation at a reasonable price and with security of tenure is a difficult one to strike. A series of Rent Acts over the years has attempted to do so: while the 1957 Act led, in some cases, to action by landlords to ensure that tenants paying controlled rent left so that new tenants could pay higher rents, the Rent Act 1965 gave tenants a degree of security of tenure and freedom from prohibitive rent rises that discouraged some landlords from letting at all. The Housing Act 1980 seeks to encourage the letting of empty property by private landlords by a new system of 'shorthold' tenancies, but it will be some years before the effect of this new Act can be evaluated.

Britain's stock of housing is getting older, and this affects all housing. The owner-occupier *tries* to keep his own home in good repair, as does the local authority. The worst housing conditions are found in the private sector, the sector which tends to house some of the most vulnerable groups within the population: the elderly living in the same place for all their adult life, and the younger and poorer members of society, whose hopes of buying, or renting from a local authority, are becoming more and more remote.

The local authority sector (commonly called council housing) is an attempt to meet a basic social need – for housing – through socially-directed means. The image of the local authority sector has tended to be authoritarian and bureaucratic, something which might change following the Housing Act 1980, which seeks to give more freedom to council tenants (eg. security of tenure, the chance to apply for grants to improve their rented property, the right for the tenure to be assigned to another member of the family when the main tenant dies, the right to buy).

The quantity and quality of housing made available by a local authority will depend on the political attitudes of the particular authority. Traditionally, Labour-controlled councils have built enthusiastically and Conservative councils reluctantly. Housing is allocated according to need, but 'need' is a term which is open to different interpretations. For example, the extent to which a local authority gives extra priority to housing applicants who have health problems varies, and community health staff should find out about allocation criteria from their local housing department in order to advise those of their clients who are in housing need. Since the Housing (Homeless Persons) Act 1977, priority in the provision of accommodation is given to certain groups, including those with children, and vulnerable groups like expectant mothers, the disabled and the elderly.

Local authorities after the war tended to go for wholesale destruction of areas of old houses with consequent loss of community networks as the small houses were replaced with large estates, often of high rise flats. This policy has resulted in problems of social isolation and vandalism in some of these estates. Since 1969, an attempt has been made to halt redevelopment on such a large scale, with rehabilitation of existing housing put forward instead. But the legacy of the past remains: large estates with good accommodation but often lacking social centres, good public transport and adequate shops — leading to problems of high maintenance costs and low morale.

Before leaving this discussion of the three main tenure groups (the housing associations have been omitted as they play such a small role in housing provision), satisfaction with housing should be mentioned. In a survey undertaken on behalf of the National Economic Development Organisation (1977) it was found that of the representative sample of 1590 people questioned, 63% who owned their housing and 52% who were buying on mortgage were very satisfied with their accommodation, compared with 33% of council and 33% of private tenants. In contrast, 2% of owners and 1% of buyers were very dissatisfied, compared with 8% of council tenants and 11% of private tenants.

Factors which influence housing

The main factors which explain the housing situation with which we are faced are changes in demand, problems of access, the effects of inflation and geographical maldistribution; these four factors are now discussed.

Changes in demand reflect the demographic changes outlined in Chapter 3. The rise in demand for housing reflects not only the absolute rise in the number of people living in the UK but also the faster rate at which separate households are formed. The elderly live longer, more unsupported mothers keep their children, and more divorce means that two households seek housing where one dwelling was previously occupied ...

Rising expectations of a separate dwelling, especially among the young, is equally relevant. Nurses used to 'live in' at the hospital during training, and often afterwards, but nowadays student nurses, like other students and other working young people, seek the freedom of accommodation of their own, perhaps competing with a family new to a town, as they search for a scarce flat in the private rented sector.

This changing pattern of demand is crucial when we turn to look at access to housing. The poor and mobile are those with the most acute problems. Those with adequate finance have no problem: houses are available to buy for those with the means to do so, assuming there is a regular salary on which the building society will usually grant a mortgage of $2\frac{1}{2}$ or 3 times its value. However, the problem varies from one area to another. The staff nurse who wished to buy a house in London would find it virtually impossible: in other areas she might find a house within her price-range. For example, the Building Societies Association (1980) has shown that in the 3rd quarter of 1979 the average price of a house in Greater London was £26,959 compared to £15,527 for a house in Yorkshire or in Humberside.

For those who cannot buy, the local authority and private rented sectors are the only options. As Figure 8.1 shows, the private rented sector is shrinking, reducing the choice and quality for ordinary families so that they can rarely find adequate accommodation at a price they can afford, and are more likely to find overcharging and poorly-maintained property the norm (outside the luxury accommodation that is available). Despite Public Health Acts and rent control, some landlords do manage to overcharge and to under-maintain their property. In a period of acute shortage, people who are desperate for any kind of accommodation are often fearful of complaining to the local Environmental Health Officer or Rent Officer in case they lose the property. One important aspect of the work of the community nurse is to encourage private tenants to use their rights in this respect.

In the local authority sector, where allocation is made according to need, waiting lists are maintained in most areas, but the way in which the waiting lists are kept and the houses are allocated varies from one local authority to another. Some local authorities have large stocks of public housing and the time on the waiting list may be short, but in Greater London, the area of the most acute housing stress in the UK, parents may watch their children spend their entire childhood in unsatisfactory conditions because they have been so long on the waiting list.

About 5% of heads of households in the UK are on local authority waiting lists, and 1% of households have another member on the waiting list. Nearly half of these are existing council tenants who wish to transfer to a different dwelling. On average, 70% of the accommodation let by local authorities is let to those on the waiting list, but in Greater London, only 54% of the new lettings go to the waiting-list applicants; of the rest, 16% go to the homeless, 13% to those displaced through slum clearance and 15% go to other people, who might include those rehoused because of their urgent health needs.

As the economic situation worsens and central government restricts local authority spending, new building in both the *private* and the *public* sectors is reduced, and this can mean that, for the poorest and most vulnerable groups and for those new to the housing market, the housing problem can only get worse. But those already housed, unless they want to move, are untouched by the housing problem.

Inflation also affects each tenure group. For the buyer the higher cost of property and increasing mortgage interest rates (from 8.5% in 1969 to 15% by 1979) make it more difficult to buy, despite the substantial advantages of ownership, ie. an asset that increases in value, as well as the tax relief on mortgage interest. In addition, whilst mortgage repayments may seem high at the beginning, they become relatively lower as incomes rise over the lifetime of the mortgage. For the private landlord inflation, rent control and high interest rates mean that it becomes more profitable to sell property and to invest the proceeds than it is to let the property and collect rents. This is an important factor in explaining the reduction in the number of private rented properties becoming available. Before the war, the tenant's rent was seen as a useful source of income to the landlord. For many landlords now, an existing tenant's rent is as nothing compared to the capital that would become available if the empty property were to be sold. For the local authority, high inflation and interest rates make the building of new housing and the conversion of older properties for rent, more expensive. Government policy, enforcing public expenditure cuts, makes even the maintenance of existing property difficult for local authorities with large stocks of old dwellings – or of new dwellings built with untried materials, whose maintenance is often becoming a new burden.

The last factor relevant to a general discussion of housing is geographical maldistribution. Demand for housing is highest in the areas of high employment; properties in areas of economic decline are easier to find, whether one is renting or buying and, of course, cheaper! This is an indicator of the inflexibility of our housing system. The redundant South Wales miner with a council flat who decided to come to London to take a job where there may be shortages of labour (eg. to be a bus conductor) would be making a good decision in terms of his job, but a disastrous decision in terms of housing: he could not buy a house in London on a bus conductor's wage, and if recognised as homeless by a local authority, he may be allocated a dwelling but one of the poorest quality: in fact, by leaving his council flat he could be considered 'intentionally homeless' and would not be allocated permanent accommodation at all.

The Housing (Homeless Persons) Act 1977 makes it the duty of local authorities to provide accommodation for homeless people who are in certain priority categories: the pregnant woman, the elderly, the family with children, a family with a disabled member. In such cases the council must provide permanent accommodation, although this might be of a lower quality than normal, and which in London may be preceded by a stay in bed-and-breakfast 'hotel' accommodation. If the Council finds that the family is 'intentionally homeless', only temporary accommodation combined with advice and assistance then needs to be provided. The line between unintentional and intentional homelessness is a fine one. Our example of a South Wales miner leaving local authority accommodation to seek work is one example of 'intentional homelessness'. Many organisations (eg. Shelter) which work to improve housing provision argue that some councils adopt too strict a definition of 'intentional', but other authorities argue that their duty to house the homeless, especially those not from the area, makes severe demands on public money. The tragedy is that if a homeless family with children is denied help under this Act, the social service department of that very same council may take those very children into care at a greater cost to the community than the offer of rented accommodation incurs, and at a greater cost to the children in terms of emotional distress. The London Boroughs deal with a disproportionate number of homeless, and those that come forward and declare themselves homeless are but the tip of an iceberg of those who are badly housed or sharing involuntarily with friends or relatives.

Yet in theory, we do in Britain have more dwellings than households! A small part of this paradox is explained by 'second homes', ie. the houses of people who live and work in towns but buy country or seaside properties for holiday use. Most of the rest of the 'surplus' is accounted for by housing that is in very poor condition and housing in areas which deter people from entry. The pattern is made more complex by the fact that the better-off are more mobile and tend to leave the central areas of cities, leaving behind those without such choices, ie. a disproportionate number of elderly, the unemployed and those families that are new to the area. The workload of the health visitor or the district nurse in an inner London Borough is very different from that of her colleague in a leafy London suburb, and the health needs of those in inner city dwellings are exacerbated by poor quality housing and difficulty in changing to something better.

Some conclusions

If the picture of the housing scene portrayed in this chapter is a complex one, this reflects reality. Housing is a jumble of private and public involvement and the ordinary person with a housing need feels oppressed and confused. During the 1970's, one positive feature has been the development of housing advice centres, run sometimes by local authorities and sometimes by voluntary bodies, which try to help people through the maze of the housing market. Another interesting phenomenon has been the growth of squatting. Often this is 'legitimate' in that the squatters have permission to use 'short life' properties, which are owned by local authorites but are in poor condition and not yet needed for their ultimate purpose, which might be slum clearance, the building of a new school or road widening. But squatting, housing advice centres, and Housing Association dwellings, all make small contributions in terms of housing supply, in a period of acute housing stress for many people.

Local authority tenure has come to be seen as 'subsidised' housing, causing some resentment amongst the more comfortably-housed owner-occupier. In fact, in 1978, the average local authority tenant was subsidised by £290 per annum, compared to £199 for each family buying its house. The private tenant's subsidy amounted to an average of £39 per annum, and as this money comes from the rent allowance scheme which helps poorer tenants to pay their rent, it reflects the fact that the poorest are found in the privately rented sector as well as in the local authority sector (where rent rebates are available to tenants unable to afford their rents).

Local authority tenants have had less control over their accommodation in the past, than even the private tenant, but security of tenure has been extended to them in the Housing Act 1980 which contains the much more controversial provision that gives local authority tenants the right to purchase their homes. In the 1979 election campaign all three major parties were committed to home ownership, but whilst council house sales were an integral part of Conservative policy (and very popular with those already in council housing which they wished to buy), the Labour Party was concerned that sales should be made only when the demand for rented housing was satisfied. Even with the opportunity to buy, the fact that about half the existing local authority tenants receive either supplementary benefit or rent rebates means that only tenants who are better off are likely to be able to purchase their dwelling.

The policy of selling council housing still relies on local authorities to implement it. Some will be hostile, including those Conservative-controlled authorities in rural areas who are frightened at the thought of council property eventually being owned by those seeking second homes. Nevertheless, even before the Act was passed, many Conservative-controlled local authorities were pressing ahead with council house sales.

The dilemma of council house sales is that the better-off council tenant in good property will want to buy and will be able to buy. The older poorer tenant, especially if in older property will not. A survey of council dwellings sold in Leeds between 1967 and 1979 (Friend 1980) showed that 4·3% of housing stock was sold but this ranged from 0·4% in an inner, poorer, part of Leeds to 9·8% of the stock in a popular suburb. The reduction in the overall amount of housing is likely to increase the time spent on the waiting list, and when allocation is made, choice will be more limited in that pleasanter and new property is likely to have been sold. This will also affect those waiting to transfer (eg. from tower block to house with garden), as the better houses are likely to be sold to existing tenants, and the flats remain within local authority ownership.

The reality is, that whatever the policy of the party in power in either central or local government, rising house prices and rising interest rates on mortgages makes a market solution to the housing problem increasingly difficult, especially for the first-time buyer, whilst public expenditure cuts are reducing the amount of new housing available to rent.

Of the social problems discussed in this book, housing remains the most difficult to describe and to solve. And within the broad, national housing problem, there are small groups of people with particularly acute housing needs that remain unmet, especially the elderly and the disabled. There is a very big shortage of sheltered accommodation with wardens, and of purpose-built accommodation, for these two groups, with consequent problems for community nursing staff and the hospital service. Overall, the elderly are *less* likely to be in local authority accommodation and to own their own home than the population at large, and sheltered accommodation is increasing too slowly to fill the gap. Hunt (1978) found 5% of the elderly people interviewed lived in sheltered accommodation with a warden (some of it provided by the social services department, some by housing departments and still other accommodation of this type provided by voluntary organistions). In addition, 3% lived in specially-built old people's accommodation, mostly local authority but again with a small contribution from the voluntary sector. But one can be sure that the cutting of local authority house building by 20% announced in 1980 (with its accompanying announcement of 20% rent rises for council tenants) will bring no comfort to those who are badly housed, old or young. It was estimated in 1976 (DoE 1977) that an additional 120,000 public homes were needed per annum! Yet housing was worst hit of all services by the public expenditure cuts of the 1970's and, indeed, in October 1980 the Secretary of State for the Environment announced that ALL further local authority expenditure on houses was to be halted indefinitely.

Radical solutions to the housing problem have been put forward. Some would argue for an end to tax relief on mortgage interest repayments, and although on grounds of equity this argument cannot be faulted, it would make any political party who proposed it automatically opposed by over 50% of the population! Another suggestion is that the cost of renting and buying should be equalised by linking both rent and repayments to the rate of inflation.

Whilst the housing situation of the vast majority of the population is good, the problem of those new to the housing market, the badly housed, the homeless, the elderly and the disabled are likely to worsen. 1980 was the year in which fewer homes were to be built than in any year since 1927 (*The Times* 1980).

References

Building Societies Association (1980) *Building Societies Association Bulletin*, No. 21. Jan.

Department of the Environment (1977) *Housing Policy: A Consultative Document*. Cmnd 6581. London: HMSO

Friend A. (1980) *A Giant Step Backwards*. London: Catholic Housing Aid Society

Hunt A. (1978) *The Elderly at Home: 1976*. OPCS. London: HMSO

National Economic Development Organisation (1977) *Degree of Satisfaction with Housing. British Market Research Bureau Housing Consumer Survey*. London: HMSO

The Times (1980) 23 April

Chapter 9

Nurses and the Welfare State

Kate Robinson

Now that we have sketched briefly some possible areas of change and progress in the welfare services, it will have become obvious that the future is uncertain. Without a doubt, the events of the past set certain limits to future activity, but within these constraints nurses can choose to respond in different ways: some may reject each and every new idea, clinging to traditional patterns of work, whilst others automatically may see any change as 'progressive' and too eagerly abandon tried and tested methods. Neither path will be appropriate in the future, compared with a middle way of testing and retaining the best of the traditional, combined with a genuine willingness to experiment with and evaluate new solutions. Changes made in any welfare system are never a 'once and for all solution' because the problems the system sets out to tackle are themselves always evolving. Planning for the future is therefore a *dynamic* process and policies must be reassessed continuously as new social data and new patterns of care become available and the economic and political context changes.

Continuous change can create great insecurity in those who are subjected to it, and many of those who experienced the reorganisation of 1974 may dread further restructuring of the NHS. However, while the slimming of the management of the NHS in the 1980's may create a stable structure for a while, changes in the process of the Service will continue. The nurse's task is twofold: firstly, to understand the context and the pressures for change in the welfare system and, secondly, to contribute effectively to the direction and management of change. To help her in these tasks is the basic rationale for this book.

There are many pressures on nursing decisions. Pressures come not only from patients or from employers but also from nurses' own aspirations for status; from ideas about appropriate financial reward; from the state of the employment market, etc. It is important, therefore, for each nurse to understand the relationship between herself and other interested parties or market forces so that her contribution to the future of nursing can represent a balanced judgement.

Two crucial areas of conflict for nurses are:

1 the relationship between health care goals and priorities and the more general goals of society;
2 the relationship between health care goals and the specifically nursing goals which shape nursing programmes.

Most nurses have a profound desire to care for people and may therefore personally sacrifice other material goals to achieve this aim. It is natural, therefore, for them to assume that giving priority to the activity of 'caring' above other possible activities is the natural and 'right' order of things. And indeed it might be so in a truly humane society, but in our society greater emphasis has been placed on other activities, such as economic expansion and increased production. For individual citizens also, spending on health care, via taxes, rather than on consumer goods, has not been as popular as might be expected in a 'civilised' community. Health care is at present only one of many activities competing for resources and nursing is only one health care activity among many.

Nurses, again because of their idealistic intentions, may come to see the goals of the health care system and those particular to nursing as the same. However, because the NHS is a *pluralistic* organisation (that is, it incorporates many different professional groups and sectors of care) many different goals and aspirations are being pursued simultaneously. Generally, some measure of agreement is reached by compromise but this means that the specifically nursing goals may sometimes be rejected or set aside.

This is true on a larger scale when a policy is made at any level, from the primary health care team to the regional health authority, but it is also important at the very lowest level of the NHS at the interface between nurse and client. The goals of the nurse may not be the same as the goals of the client, and the nurse must be sensitive to the need to reach a compromise between the client's wishes and her duties as a state employee in addition to her responsibilities to her profession. Some nurses see no conflict here – believing that they are always on the side of the patient – but there must always be a potential conflict when care is provided by the community for the individual.

This conflict sometimes involves the material provision of care, that is, 'is there enough of it and is it of the right sort?', and every nurse who has discharged a patient before he wanted to go home because 'we need the beds' has experienced this problem. However, with increasing cutbacks in spending in the NHS, this conflict will become more acute. Some nurses have already taken collective action in conjunction with other hospital workers to maintain services to patients against the instructions of management, either by 'sit-ins' or 'work-ins'. Obviously, these nurses believe either that the interests of the patient deserved primacy over the wishes of the community or that the community did not understand the implications of its decisions.

The conflict between individual and community interests may be ethical as well as material in areas such as child welfare, where the community now reserves the right to set minimum standards of child care and attempts to enforce them through welfare agencies, including health visitors. Similarly, the district nurse may find pressures coming from the community, say, to remove an elderly man from his own home. The request may be presented as being for the old man's own good, but the reality is often that the community – family, friends, and neighbours – wants to be rid of the burden and embarrassment of having an 'incompetent' person in their midst. How far should society set standards of incompetence and should it enforce them through the intervention of medical or nursing staff?

In every area of care, therefore, there is a potential conflict between the nurse, other welfare workers, the client, the family, and the community. It is important to re-emphasise that these are not merely areas of conflict for negotiation by the professional body or trade union; they exist for each individual nurse. Every practising nurse is a member of the nursing profession, an employee, a citizen, and a potential patient. The values and goals appropriate to each role may be different, and an understanding of these differences will enable each nurse to contribute effectively to the debate on the future of the health service and of nursing. Each of these roles has a different means of expression: professional aspirations via a professional association; employment problems via a trade union;

citizens' rights and responsibilities through lay democratic channels of local and national government. Any nurse can choose to use some channels or none at all, but as several channels exist by which she can influence the future, any abdication of the responsibility of democratic action rather forfeits the right to complain about developments later on.

Professional associations

The major professional association claiming to represent all aspects of nursing is the Royal College of Nursing, but other organisations such as the Royal College of Midwives and the Health Visitors Association represent particular spheres of activity. Many professional associations also function as trade unions and are officially certified as such under the Trades Unions and Labour Relations Acts 1974 and 1976.

The professional association is, according to Merton (1958) '... an organisation of practitioners who judge one another as professionally competent and who have banded together to perform social functions which they cannot perform in their separate capacity as individuals'. Unlike trade unions, professional associations profess to promote the interests of the professions as a whole and of the community, as well as those of individual practitioners.

Professional associations operate in two directions – externally and internally. Externally, they relate to government and official bodies and act as an adviser on matters of policy relating to the profession and as a pressure group to promote the interests of the profession; internally, they offer a range of services to their members which includes educational programmes, setting standards for practice and ethics, professional indemnity insurance and legal and professional advisory services.

Because the professional association is concerned with the progress of the profession as a whole, its attention is likely to be focused on the frontiers of change where practical and ethical problems will be most acute. It is interesting, for instance, to study the activities of the Societies of the Royal College of Nursing, which currently function in the fields of geriatric nursing, occupational health, oncology nursing, primary health care, psychiatric nursing, and research.

Although a professional association can greatly facilitate education and research to improve professional practice, its influence can also inhibit progress. A commitment to professionalism implies a commitment to the exclusivity of a body of knowledge which only its members have mastered. Such exclusivity in nursing knowledge, as in other fields, may not be conductive to the kind of public debates about practice or the kind of client autonomy which many wish to see developed in the NHS.

Similarly, the professional association may feel committed to the expansion of the areas of expertise or control enjoyed by its members, and certainly might oppose any diminution of the profession's sphere of activity. Just as some doctors have resented the loss of some areas of activity to nurses, so nurses in turn may resent the loss of activities or client groups to operating department assistants or social workers. Professionalisation could greatly threaten the kind of flexibility in allocating tasks and client groups that was advocated by the Royal Commission. 'The interface between the health and social services is more sharply drawn (or the opportunity of successfully blurring it lost) by the development of professional consciousness and competitiveness.' (Willcocks 1979).

The potential conflict between the needs of individual nurses, the nursing profession and the community is well illustrated by the debate which followed the publication of the Jay Report (1979). This report advocated a philosophy of and approach to the care of mentally handicapped people with which few nurses would have disagreed; but, because it recommended, as the means of achieving this aim, a system in which the traditional professional carers (ie. nurses) would have been replaced by a 'new' professional group whose preparation and practice would be controlled by social worker rather than nursing institutions, the report was strongly opposed by all the nursing organisations, to such an extent that debate about the 'model of care' was completely submerged beneath the fight to retain mental handicap nursing as a nursing specialty and to protect the position of those nurses at present working in this field.

Basically, the professional association acts on the belief that what is good for the profession is good for the public, but Merton told American nurses many years ago (1958) that '... at least in the short run, it is not the case that what is good for the profession of medicine or of law or of nursing is necessarily best for the community, or conversely'. Other writers have gone further. Shaw's view that '... all professions are conspiracies against the laity' (*The Doctor's Dilemma*, Act I) and Illich's account of *Medical Nemesis* (1975) are perhaps the best known, but more recently (1979) Garner, for example, has argued that the most fundamental dilemma facing any health service is '... the fact that the interests of medicine and the interests of a health service are not one and the same'. These writers were specifically concerned with the medical profession but the point is equally valid for other occupational groups, including nurses.

Trade unions

The principal organisations performing an exclusively trade union function in the NHS on behalf of nurses are the Confederation of Health Service Employees (COHSE), the National Union of Public Employees (NUPE) and the National Association of Local Government Officers (NALGO).

Although there is a tradition among British trade unions that they exist solely to further the material interests of their members and do not directly engage in broader political issues, any trade union acting for NHS employees will obviously have a direct interest in government policy relating to public expenditure. The trade unions have therefore become involved both directly and through the Trades Union Congress in discussions on the general future of the health service. Because their membership includes other occupations besides nursing, they have an interest in the balance between occupational groups employed in the NHS as well as simply the numbers of nursing jobs.

As unions have the primary function of protecting members' jobs through any legal means, they may choose to combat any action of their employers by instructing their members to withdraw their labour. Because the labour of nurses directly involves the welfare of patients and not the manufacture of goods this poses both an ethical and a practical problem. Ethically, the problem is that any industrial action may bring harm to the patient, whose interests the nurse purports to serve and, practically, it does not directly alter the prospects of the employer, except, paradoxically, by saving money! These problems are particularly acute in the community where the withdrawal of nursing services does not even have the dramatic impact on public opinion that the closure of an acute hospital might have.

Professional bodies are particularly reluctant to use the weapon of industrial action, overtly because of the notion of service to the public that they seek to promote. However, it must be said that most professions have had the ability to secure more than adequate remuneration by other means and have not needed to resort to withdrawal of labour or similar activity. When they feel that their control over their work situation is threatened they have been prepared to use more militant methods; doctors, for instance, have repeatedly threatened to withdraw their labour from the NHS since its inception and have generally had their own way as a consequence. In the 1970's, for example, junior hospital doctors took industrial action over pay and conditions, and consultants also restricted their working in protest action over the availability of pay beds (which directly affects their pay and conditions).

In 1979, and again in 1980, the RCN membership confirmed its long-established policy against the use of industrial action in furtherance of a pay claim, and the trade unions involved in the pay dispute of 1979-80 adopted a voluntary code of action to protect patients' interests during industrial action. COHSE issued a statement defending the right to take industrial action, including withdrawal of labour, but also stated that '. . . when operating restrictive measures, a reasonable standard of patient care will be maintained and the respect for human dignity . . . will be observed'. There was at the time considerable discussion of withdrawing the right to strike from NHS employees. However, such a legal restraint applies only to the police and the armed forces and it seems likely that any attempt to extend this policy to other occupational groups would be bitterly opposed by the trade union movement as a whole – whose members fought hard and sometimes bloody battles for the rights workers now enjoy. It would in any case be an extremely difficult ban to enforce amongst all NHS workers.

The debate about the nurse's right to strike was brought to a head in 1979 when the General Nursing Council issued a statement that a nurse would have '. . . a case to answer on the score of professional misconduct' if she '. . . puts the health, safety or welfare of her patients at risk by taking strike or other industrial action . . . just as by any other action on his or her part' (GNC 1979). Trade unions such as COHSE and NUPE attacked the statement as '... intimidation and blackmail'; the professional associations accepted it as '... simply a statement about professional responsibility, a reminder of a fact which some people would prefer to forget – that those who choose to become members of a profession thereby accept certain rights and responsibilities which are not laid upon other people' (Clark 1979). The debate was well presented at the time in a series of articles (Nursing Mirror 1979) by leaders of the major professional organisations and trade unions, but clearly the conflict between the nurse as a professional and as an employee like any other employee has still to be resolved.

Joint Staff Consultative Committees

The management arrangements for the reorganised health service in 1974 included machinery for consultation and negotiation (excluding subjects negotiated by the Whitley Council) between staff and management at local level; committees were established at district, area and regional level. Such committees will work only if both sides are prepared genuinely to consult and discuss with open minds, and the staff side must truly represent the staff and maintain good channels for communication with those they represent.

There has been, in the past, some reluctance on the part of professional workers to consult and negotiate with other manual and white-collar workers in the health services. In evidence to the Royal Commission on the NHS (1979) the TUC remarked: 'In the NHS this principle (industrial democracy) has applied in the past only to doctors and nurses, and the supporting staff on which the Service is heavily dependent have largely been ignored' (TUC undated). Within the Joint Staff Consultative Committee all occupational groups have the opportunity to participate through membership of recognised trade unions. In some areas, however, a dispute between TUC-affiliated unions and other unions has led to the withdrawal of the former group from JSCCs and the establishment of a separate consultative machinery.

The ACAS evidence to the Royal Commission was critical of both management and unions in the NHS, and concluded that a comprehensive overhaul of the industrial relations policy was overdue. In particular, local negotiating machinery was felt to be inadequate, perhaps because in the past the NHS had relied too greatly on the goodwill of the workforce. The Royal Commission endorsed this criticism and, as with so many other facets of change, stressed the importance of adequate education: 'The health departments and staff organisations should give urgent attention to industrial relations training for both staff representatives and management' (Recommendation 59).

Like it or not – and many nurses do not like it – industrial relations within the health service has become an important determinant of health service policy, particularly at local level. Nurses are being forced to become more conscious of their role as workers in the NHS.

The nurse as an independent expert

There are two other notable ways by which the voice of nurses is heard in the NHS, namely, through the professional advisory machinery, and through membership of the health authorities themselves.

Professional advisory committees   Within each area and region there are professional advisory committees, including a Nursing and Midwifery Advisory Committee, whose function is to advise the health authority (AHA or RHA) on matters relating to the various spheres of professional activity. This advice is independent of and in addition to the advice which the authority receives from its nurse officers (the DNO, ANO and RNO). The members of the Nursing and Midwifery Advisory Committee are qualified nurses working as practitioners in the various specialties of nursing within the NHS and elected directly by their nursing colleagues.

These committees function much more successfully in some areas than in others. Difficulty in establishing election procedures and the low level of participation by nurses in some areas has led some people to doubt their value, and the consultative document *Patients First* (1979) specifically raises the question of the need for their review. It would be a tragedy if such an important channel for the nurse's influence were to be lost by default; the best defence, however, is evidence that more nurses are actually using them.

Membership of health authorities   Members of health authorities are appointed and not elected, but in making appointments the Secretary of State and the Regional Authority (the appointing agents) take into account nominations received from relevant groups and from individuals. Members are appointed as individuals, not representatives (except for local government representatives – see Chapter 6), and for the contribution that each can make as an individual. In this way, a nurse is as eligible for appointment as a solicitor or a carpenter, but, in addition, one place is reserved specifically for a nurse member. The appointment is likely to reflect the nominations received from local nursing organisations, but the nurse, if she can be regarded as a representative at all, represents nursing rather than nurses. Membership of a health authority gives a direct say in the determination of health service policy at local level, and the nurse member can be a very influential champion of nursing, especially if she is well briefed by her nursing colleagues, and is not afraid to present the nursing view with force when necessary.

The nurse as a citizen

It is impossible to include in this short book a full discussion of all the democratic channels which are open to the nurse as an ordinary citizen, but we can emphasise a nurse's responsibility to ensure that all democratic discussions and decisions about the health service are informed discussions and decisions. A nurse can use any of the routes of influence described above, but can also speak as an informed citizen about the problems of nursing and health care, provided that she makes clear that she speaks only as an individual and not as a representative or delegate of other nurses.

There are many organisations – political parties, local pressure groups, voluntary organisations, etc. – which require and would welcome specialised advice. Some of these organisations may be specifically related to the NHS, for instance a nurse might serve on a Community Health Council or be actively involved in a charity providing funds and support to the NHS. But other organisations can also benefit from an input of health expertise: tenants' associations need to know about safety hazards, youth groups need people with counselling skills.

At present, no nurse sits as a Member of Parliament in the House of Commons, although there is one nurse, Baroness McFarlane of Llandaff, in the House of Lords. A few nurses, however, are active in the political parties at local level, and in local government. Nurses who serve as local councillors can bring their expertise to bear on many topics: the environment, social services, planning, etc., and as Elizabeth Day, nurse, health visitor and district councillor, points out: 'If local authorities do not appear to be interested in the total concept of health the blame lies with the apathy and disinterest of local health workers, who take no interest in local affairs, nor lobby their elected members at all levels of government' (*Nursing Times* 1980). Indeed, participation in such political activities will probably be of benefit to the nurse as her views and opinions will have to be tested against the direct competition of the views and opinions of others, and she will be able to see her proposals in a wider perspective.

All nurses have views on non-nursing matters of government policy – rates, taxes, foreign affairs, the list is endless – many of which will be in direct conflict with nursing aspirations. This conflict became more acute as the apparent consensus politics of the 1960's and 1970's, when there was some measure of agreement on suitable levels of welfare spending, gave way to sharp divisions over government spending and the role of the state. As a citizen, a nurse may vote for lower taxes and consequent cutbacks in public spending; as an employee, the same nurse will resent uncertainty about her employment prospects and career opportunities; as a professional, the nurse is likely to oppose reductions in services to patients and the abandonment of programmes of education and innovative schemes.

The difficulties encountered in coping with change in the NHS are both a product of and also contribute to low staff morale. The Royal Commission (1979) commented on the poor morale found among health service employees and pinpointed four contributing factors:

    1 the short-term effects of reorganisation;
    2 the country's economic difficulties;
    3 changing roles and relationships;
    4 criticisms of the NHS.

It will be obvious from the discussion in previous chapters that none of these factors is likely to disappear, and although the reorganisation of 1974 is now firmly in the past, the planned reorganisation for 1982 is also engendering insecurity.

Although, as we have seen, the nurse has many channels of influence open to her, she may not be using them as creatively or as positively as might be wished. There are many reasons for this, but perhaps two can be pinpointed. Firstly, some nurses consider that it is not quite 'nice' to take part in political activities. Traditionally, nurses are expected to be docile and compliant, avoiding confrontation and conflict, and are reluctant to assume authority other than in specific areas (Leininger 1974). These attitudes have arisen not only because of the historical pattern of hospital nursing being ancilliary to the medical profession, but also because most nurses, at least in the general nursing sector, have been women and therefore subject to the cultural expectation that women lack initiative, authority, and management skills. Secondly, the proliferation of channels of influence has led to confusion, and hence to apathy. A Study Group (Kings Fund Centre 1976) set up to investigate whether clinically-based nurses were prepared to participate actively in democratic channels and had the tools to do so, found that nurses needed extra training in many aspects of decision making, eg. how to work on committees, how to research areas of policy, etc. However, three of the recommendations are particularly relevant to this book: they are that nurses should have a clear understanding of

1 what is meant by the terms used, eg. policy making, strategic planning, participative management, representative, confidential;
2 the ways in which the nursing service interlocks and is interdependent with other services; and .
3 developing social, economic, and political trends and how they affect the service.

We hope that after reading this book the nurse is at least better informed and is able to participate fully in building the new welfare services of the 1980's: but the place of the nursing services in the welfare sphere still depends on the willingness of each nurse to act creatively, to co-operate with other welfare workers, but always to remember the purpose of this huge welfare edifice we have described – to serve the client.

References

Clark J. (1979) *Nursing Mirror*, 16, 23 & 30 Aug.

Day E. (1980) *Nursing Times*, 3 April

DHSS (1979) *Patients First: A Consultative Paper on the Structure and Management of the NHS in England and Wales*. London: HMSO

Garner L. (1979) *The NHS: Your Money or Your Life*. Harmondsworth: Penguin

Illich I. (1975) *Medical Nemesis*. London: Calder & Boyars

King Edward's Hospital Fund for London (1976) *Nurses in Committee: Study Group and Guidelines*. London: King's Fund Centre

Leininger L. (1974) The leadership crisis in nursing: a critical problem and challenge. *Journal of Nursing Administration*, March/April

Merton R. K. (1958) The functions of the professional association. *American Journal of Nursing*, **58**(1)

Report of the Committee of Enquiry into Mental handicap Nursing and Care (1979) (Jay Report) Cmnd 7468, I & II. London: HMSO

Royal Commission on the National Health Service (Chairman: Sir Alec Merrison) (1979) *Report*. Cmnd 7615. London: HMSO

Willcocks A. (1979) Weakness of consultation. *Health and Social Services Journal*, 27 April

Essential Reading

The following books contain very detailed descriptions of the range of health and social services provided by statutory and voluntary bodies in Britain. The latest edition is given here, but it should be noted that these books are regularly revised.

Davies B. M. (1980) *Community Health, Preventive Medicine and Social Services*. London: Bailliere Tindall

Family Welfare Association (1980) *Guide to the Social Services*. (1980). London: Family Welfare Association

Wilmott P. (1978) *Consumer's Guide to the British Social Services*. Harmondsworth: Penguin Books

Recommended further reading

Atkinson P., Dingwall R. & Murcott A. (1979) *Prospects for the National Health*. London: Croom Helm

Brearley P. *et al.* (1978) *The Social Context of Health Care*. London: Martin Robertson/Oxford: Basil Blackwell

Brown R. G. S. (1975) *The Management of Welfare*. London: Fontana

Central Office of Information (1977) *Social Security in Britain: Reference Pamphlet 90*. London: HMSO

Doyal L. (1979) *The Political Economy of Health*. London: Pluto Press

Royal Commission on the National Health Service (Chairman: Sir Alec Merrison) (1979) *Report*. Cmnd. London: HMSO
OR
A Source for Patients: Conclusions and Recommendations of the Royal Commission's Report. London: HMSO

DHSS (1979) *Patients First: A Consultative Paper on the Structure and Management of the NHS in England and Wales*. London: HMSO

Holman R. (1978) *Poverty: Explanations of Social Deprivation*. London: Martin Robertson

Judge K. (1978) *Rationing Social Services*. London: Heinemann

Lancaster A. (1979) *Nursing and Midwifery Sourcebook*. London: Allen & Unwin/Beaconsfield Publishers

Sleeman J. (1979) *Resources for the Welfare State*. London: Longmans

Titmuss R. (1974) *Social Policy: An Introduction*. London: Allen & Unwin

Townsend P. (1979) *Poverty in the United Kingdom*. Harmondsworth: Penguin

Watkin B. (1978) *The National Health Service: The First Phase 1948–74 and After*. London: Allen & Unwin

Widgery D. (1979) *Health in Danger: The Crisis in the National Health Service*. London: Macmillan

Useful Addresses

STATUTORY ORGANISATIONS
  National
Department of Education and Science: Elizabeth House, York Road,
  London SE1
Department of the Environment: 2 Marsham Street, London SW1
Department of Health and Social Security: Alexander Fleming House,
  Elephant & Castle, London SE1 (local offices dealing with National
  Insurance and Supplementary Benefits listed in local telephone book
  under 'Health and Social Security').
*Parliamentary Commissioner for Administration and for the Health
  Service:* Church House, Great Smith Street, London SW1
Scottish Home and Health Department: St Andrews House, Edinburgh
  EH1 3DE
Welsh Office (Health and Social Work Department): Pearl Assurance
  House, Greyfriars Road, Cardiff

  Local
Social Services Departments: Listed in local telephone book under the
  appropriate local authority

PROFESSIONAL ORGANISATIONS

British Association of Social Workers: 16 Kent Street, Birmingham 5
British Medical Association: BMA House, Tavistock Square, London
  WC1H 9TP
Central Midwives Board: 39 Harrington Gardens, London SW7 4JY
Confederation of Health Service Employees: Glen House, High Street,
  Banstead, Surrey
Council for the Education and Training of Health Visitors: Clifton House,
  Euston Road, London NW1 2RS
General Nursing Council for England and Wales: 23 Portland Place,
  London W1A 1BA
Health Visitors Association: 36 Eccleston Square, London SW1
National Association of Local Government Officers: 1 Mabledon Place,
  London WC1

161

National Association of Public Employees: 8 Aberdeen Terrace, London SE3

Queen's Nursing Institute: 57 Lower Belgrave Street, London SW 1 0LR

Royal College of Midwives: 15 Mansfield Street, London W 1M 0BE

Royal College of Nursing: Henrietta Place, London W 1M 0AB

VOLUNTARY ORGANISATIONS

Age Concern: 60 Pitcairn Road, Mitcham, Surrey

Child Poverty Action Group: 1 Macklin Street, London WC2

Disablement Income Group: Attlee House, Toynbee Hall, Commercial Street, London E 1

Family Welfare Association: 501–503 Kingsland Road, London E8

King's Fund Centre and Library: 126 Albert Street, London NW 1

MIND (National Association for Mental Health): 22 Harley Street, London W 1N 2ED

National Association for the Welfare of Children in Hospital: 7 Exton Street, London SE 1

National Children's Bureau: 8 Wakley Street, London EC1V 7QE

National Council for One-Parent Families: 255 Kentish Town Road, London NW5 2LX

National Council for Voluntary Organisations (formerly National Council for Social Service): 26 Bedford Square, London WC1B 3HU

National Society for Mentally Handicapped Children: Pembridge Hall, Pembridge Square, London W 2

National Society for the Prevention of Cruelty to Children: 1 Riding House Street, London W 1P 8AA

Northern Ireland Council of Social Service: 2 Annandale Avenue, Belfast BT7 3JR

Royal Association for Disability and Rehabilitation (Radar): 25 Mortimer Street, London W 1

Royal National Institute for the Blind: 224 Great Portland Street, London W 1

Scottish Association for Mental Health: 18-19 Claremont Crescent, Edinburgh EH7 4QT

Scottish Council for Single Parents: 44 Albany Street, Edinburgh EH 1 3QR

Scottish Council for Social Service: 18-19 Claremont Street, Edinburgh EH7 4QT

Shelter: 86 The Strand, London WC2

Index

AREA HEALTH AUTHORITIES,
94–97, 156

BEVERIDGE REPORT, 36–37, 61,
68, 86
five giants, 36, 37
Briggs Report, 9, 10
British Association of Social
Workers, 10
British Medical Association, 8, 9

CABINET, 5–7
Case conference, 101, 130
Central government, 4–6, 12,
41–44
Charges in the NHS, 41, 44, 51, 55,
56–57, 72
Child Benefit, 69, 78
Child health services, 86
Child minding, 3
Children, social service provision
for, 116, 121–2, 130–132
Childrens Acts 1948, 1963, 1969,
1970, 121
Childrens Act 1980, 122
Chronically Sick and Disabled Act
1970, 8, 120–121
Civil Service, 5, 6, 8, 11
Collaboration, 82, 100–103, 126,
128–133
Committees of enquiry, 9, 92,
105–106
Community care, 91–93, 103, 123,
131

Community Health Councils, 94,
96, 104–107, 109
Confederation of Health Service
Employees COHSE, 8, 10,
152–4
Conservative Party, 33, 38–39, 41
Court Report, 10, 86

DAY NURSERIES, 3, 35
Demography see population,
Dentists, 97
Department of Health & Social
Security DHSS, 4–6, 98, 111,
127
Disabled, 16, 37, 70–72, 99, 116,
121, 145–146
Disabled Income Group DIG, 8, 71
Disability Alliance, 10
District/District Management
Teams, 94, 96, 98, 100
District General Hospital, 93
District Health Authority, 108–110
District Nurse, 83, 92, 101, 132
District Planning Team, 129
Doctors, 9, 23, 30, 56, 89, 96,
100–104, 111–112, 130, 132,
153
Drugs, cost of, 57

EDUCATION, 20, 36, 41–43, 51, 59
Elderly, 33–34, 37, 55, 64, 67,
91–2, 99, 116–117, 121, 128,
131, 145–146
Ely Hospital, 92, 105

FAMILY, 34, 64, 67, 74, 92, 123–124
Family Allowances, 37, 69
Family Income Supplement, 63, 70, 73
Family Practitioner Committee, 100–103, 106, 109
Farleigh Hospital, 92, 106

GENERAL NURSING COUNCIL, 153–154
General practitioners, 57, 89, 96, 100–103, 130

HEALTH ADVISORY SERVICE, 105
Health Care Planning Team, 100, 129
Health centre, 101
Health services, 11, 20, 81, 83–4, 93
Health Services and Public Health Act 1968, 121
Health visitor, 82–3, 101, 130
Health Visitors Association, 10, 150
Home helps, 116, 117
Homeless, 137, 142–143
Homelessness, intentional, 142
Hospitals, 51, 57, 88–90, 91, 93, 97, 99, 131
Hospital Advisory Service, 105
Housing, 20, 37, 47, 53, 63, 136–146
Housing Advice Centres, 142–143
Housing Act 1980, 138
Housing (Homeless Persons) Act 1980, 142
Housing associations, 139, 144

INDUSTRIAL RELATIONS IN THE NHS, 97, 103–104, 154–155
Industrial Injuries Scheme, 69
Inequalities in health care, 97–100
Intermediate treatment, 121–122

JAY REPORT (ON MENTAL HANDICAP NURSING), 151
Joint Consultative Committees, 96, 102–103, 108, 129
Joint Care Planning Team, 103–104
Joint financing, 102–103
Joint Staff Consultative Committees, 154

LABOUR PARTY, 28, 33, 38–39, 41, 43
Liberal Party, 28, 33, 38, 40
Local authority housing, 136–139, 141, 144–145
Local government, 11–15, 41–44, 88, 116, 126

MEALS ON WHEELS, 92, 116–7, 128
Means-tested benefits, 72
Medical care, 82
Mentally handicapped, provisions for the, 92, 99, 117, 122
Mental Health Act 1959, 123
Mentally ill, provisions for the, 51, 99, 122
Midwives, 30, 101
MIND see National Association for Mental Health, 10–11
Minister of Health, 88
Morbidity, 90
Mortality, 86, 90
Mortgage tax relief, 47, 53, 137, 141

NATIONAL ASSISTANCE, 61
National Assistance Act 1948, 37, 121
National Association of Local Government Officers NALGO, 10, 152

National Association for Mental
     Health MIND, 10–11
National Health Service, 3–8,
     11–12, 16–19, 23, 81–115,
     147
   Act 1944, 37
   Act 1980, 107
   charges, 41, 55, 57, 72
   and complaints, 106–107
   expenditure, 11, 51, 55, 57, 84
   organisation in Scotland, Wales
     & N Ireland, 83
   reorganisation, 88–97, 107–110,
     158
   resource allocation, 87, 97–99
   and trade unions, 10, 154–155
   see also industrial relations;
     public expenditure; Royal
     Commission on the NHS
National Insurance, 37, 48, 53, 61,
     68, 70–71, 73
National Union of Public
     Employees NUPE, 10, 152
Non-accidental injury, 130–132
Normansfield Hospital Enquiry,
     105–6
Nurses, 9, 17–18, 23, 43–4, 60, 81,
     99, 104, 112, 132, 147–159
   as citizens, 156–7
   and health service
     administration, 96, 156
   and trade unions, 152–154
Nursing, 30, 148
   in the community, 92, 97, 101,
     132
   the mentally handicapped, 151
   as a profession, 30
Nursing and Midwifery Advisory
     Committee, 96, 155

OMBUDSMAN see Parliamentary
     Commissioner for Health, 106
One-parent family, 64, 67

Owner-occupied housing, 136

PARLIAMENT, 4–5, 6–8, 12, 24, 37,
     110
Parliamentary Commissioner for
     Health, 106
Patients, 81, 99, 104–106, 147
Patients' Association, 8
Patients First, 97, 107, 109
Pensions, 29, 48
Personal social services, 20, 51,
     81–83
Physically handicapped see
     disabled,
Political parties, 4, 6–8, 33, 38–44
Population, 34, 91, 120, 140
Poverty, 16, 24, 27, 35, 61–73, 75
Pressure groups, 7–8, 10–12, 15,
     110, 112
Preventive medicine, 86–87, 91
Prime Minister, 4, 6
Private landlords, 136–138,
     140–141
Professional organisations, 30,
     110–11, 149, 153
Public expenditure, 7–8, 16, 23–24,
     33, 35, 37, 39–48, 50, 52–54,
     99, 119, 122
   effects of cuts on, 43–44, 93,
     132–133, 145–146, 149
   on health, 3, 7, 11–12, 48, 50, 58,
     84
   on housing, 46, 141–2
   on personal social services, 48,
     127
   on social services, 117, 122

RATES, 12, 51
Referral to social service
     departments, 130
Regional Allocation Working Party
     RAWP, 54, 98, 110
Regional health authority, 94, 98

Rent Acts 1957, 1965, 138
Rent officer, 140
Report of the Committee on Nursing (Briggs Report), 9, 10
Report of the Committee on Local Authority and Allied Personal Social Services (Seebohm Report, 9, 116, 119
Residential care, 37, 55, 116–117, 121, 123
Royal College of Midwives, 10, 150
Royal College of Nursing, 8, 10, 150, 153–154
Royal Commission on Mental Health 1959, 92
Royal Commission on the NHS, 17, 29, 51, 56–58, 86, 97, 108–109, 157
Royal Commissions, 9

SEEBOHM REPORT, 9, 116, 119
Secretary of State for the Social Services, 81, 105
Sheltered accommodation, 8, 136
Social class, 86–87, 111
Social Security, 20, 23, 29, 37, 61, 70–75
  benefits outlined, 75–79
Social Security Act 1980, 74
Social Security (Pensions) Act 1975, 69–70
Social Security Advisory Committee, 74
Social Services, 16, 23, 29, 33, 54, 58–61, 82, 117

expenditure, 46–48, 117, 120, 122, 126–127
Social Services Act 1970, 9, 129
Social Services Committee, 81
Social services departments, 15, 17, 81–82, 93, 102, 119–120, 125–126, 143
Social workers, 17, 23, 82–83, 92, 101, 112, 117, 119–120, 122, 131
Supplementary Benefits, 53, 61–63, 71–74

TAXATION, 2, 40–41, 47, 79
Trade unions, 7, 103–4, 149, 152–154
Treasury, 6

UNEMPLOYED, 16, 20

VOLUNTARY ORGANISATIONS, 3, 23, 81, 117, 122–127, 142, 143
Volunteers, 124–126

WELFARE STATE, 16, 20–28, 30, 37, 39, 44, 61–63
Whitley Council, 154
Whittington Hospital Enquiry, 92, 106
Women, changing position of, 34
  family role of, 36
  and marriage, 35
  and work, 35
  traditional role of, 158